The International Library of Psychology

CHILDHOOD AND AFTER

T0264538

Founded by C. K. Ogden

The International Library of Psychology

PSYCHOANALYSIS
In 28 Volumes

CHILDHOOD AND AFTER

Some Essays and Clinical Studies

SUSAN ISAACS

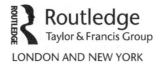

Routledge
Taylor & Francis Group

LONDON AND NEW YORK

First published in 1948
by Routledge
2 Park Square, Milton Park, Abingdon, Oxfordshire OX14 4RN
711 Third Avenue, New York, NY 10017

First issued in paperback 2014

Routledge is an imprint of the Taylor and Francis Group, an informa business

British Library Cataloguing in Publication Data
A CIP catalogue record for this book
is available from the British Library

Childhood and After
ISBN 0415-21100-X
Psychoanalysis: 28 Volumes
ISBN 0415-21132-8
The International Library of Psychology: 204 Volumes
ISBN 0415-19132-7

ISBN 13: 978-1-138-87564-7 (pbk)
ISBN 13: 978-0-415-21100-0 (hbk)

CONTENTS

PREFACE

THIS volume does not include all the papers published by me during the period covered, but consists partly of a selection of technical psycho-analytical studies, partly of papers which either touch upon the bearing of psycho-analysis on the upbringing and education of young children, or link their social and emotional life with their intellectual and practical needs.

Most of these essays deal with children; in any case they rest upon the relationship between childhood and adult life, as for example "The Modifications of the Ego", where it can be clearly seen that it is not possible to understand the adult without going back to the feelings, phantasies and experiences of the infant. In "The Criteria of Interpretation" there is very little reference to children, the paper being concerned with psycho-analytic work with adults, but the same implications will be seen there also.

In the nature of the case some of the essays are more popular than others, but I hope that none of them will be found so technical as to be devoid of interest to those concerned with the psychological problems of little children. Those previously published have not been changed save for a few minor verbal alterations. They are arranged simply in order of publication (or delivery, if previously unpublished).

November 1947.   SUSAN ISAACS.

ACKNOWLEDGMENTS

I WISH to express my indebtedness to the many friends who have helped me in preparing this volume for the press: in particular to Mrs. Melanie Klein, Dr. Paula Heimann and Mrs. Joan Riviere, as regards the psycho-analytical papers previously unpublished; also to Miss Dorothy E. M. Gardner and Dr. Evelyn Lawrence. Their help has been generous and invaluable. To Mrs. Klein and Mrs. Riviere I owe an immense debt for twenty years' teaching and inspiration, one which never can be repaid. From my husband, too, I have had constant support and the most helpful criticism in the original writing of the essays, and in their preparation for the press.

Furthermore, for permission to republish certain of the essays, acknowledgments are due to:

The British Journal of Medical Psychology,
The International Journal of Psycho-Analysis,
The Nursery School Association,
The New Education Fellowship, and the
Education Section of the British Psychological Society.

SUSAN ISAACS.

November, 1947.

I

THE MENTAL HYGIENE OF THE PRE-SCHOOL CHILD[1],[2]

(1928)

It will, I suppose, be agreed that no subject of greater psycho-logical interest or practical importance could come before this Society than that of mental hygiene in the little child. As with disease in general, attention has within the last few years shifted from the problem of cure to that of prevention; and this has come to mean, here perhaps more than anywhere, a corresponding shift of interest from the adult to the child, and from the child to the infant. Whether as doctors, social observers or educators, all those who have any concern with the neurotic adult, or with any disturbances of conduct and mental health in youth or manhood, are now developing an interest in the early disposing factors, and possible ways of dealing with these. The intelligent parent is asking for advice as to what he should do to avoid neurosis—if there be anything *to* be done; and here and there he meets with those who speak with no uncertain voice as to what should be done and what should be left undone. Others of us who have had opportunities of studying both neurotic and normal children at close hand over a long period, and in the light of some knowledge of their parents' minds and home conditions, are more sensible of the obscurities of the problem, and of the difficulties of laying down any broad body of clear and definite principles of certain prophylaxis, in the present state of our knowledge. We know much, but by no means all, nor with complete certainty.

I should like to consider some of the difficulties in the way of setting out clear lines of advice for the prevention of neurosis— whether to this or that parent, or as general social and educational doctrine, bearing on the mental hygiene of the pre-school child.

If, then, we have come to look for the point of origin of neurosis in early childhood, the first question clearly is how to know the

---

[1] Being a paper read at a joint meeting of the Educational and the Medical Sections of the British Psychological Society on June 27th, 1928.

[2] *British Journal of Medical Psychology*, Vol. VIII, Pt. 3, 1928.

neurotic child, or the neurotic-child-to-be, when we see him.

In many cases that is, of course, easy enough. If a child of, say, five or six years has persistent night-terrors, or enuresis; if he masturbates constantly; if he is patently and continually destructive and defiant, stealing, biting, behaving with marked cruelty to younger children; if he is excessively clinging and querulous, if he shows overt anxieties and phobias, or marked speech disturbances such as stammering or refusal to try to talk at a late age—in any of these situations it is easy enough to affix the label of neurotic. The physician will do it at once, and nowadays many a well-informed parent is able to. But it will, I think, be agreed that in these very cases it is hardly any longer a matter of prophylaxis, but already one of well-developed neurosis. If one approaches the problem in a stereotyped way from the point of view of the grown-up, then of course anything that happens in the years under six might be held to be an "early" stage of development and disease; and anything that is done to alleviate matters might be considered prophylactic. But that is to give a naïve value to the mere passage of time which it does not deserve. All our knowledge of genetic psychology in general, and of the nature of neurosis in particular, runs counter to such a view. The analysis of adults shows that the pattern of their responses was already firm by the end of the period we are considering, the rest of their development being very largely an embroidery around the original theme. But particularly is this true of the neurotic, since a certain fixity of response, a way of forcing all later experience into the mould of the earlier, is one of the essential characters of neurosis. Young as the child may be in years, the psychology of the neurosis compels us to regard such manifest difficulties as those mentioned as signs of definite and matured neurosis; and the problem in these cases as already one of cure, not prevention.

For preventive mental hygiene, our signs must needs be more delicate and earlier seen.

Unfortunately, we have so far hardly any comparative data upon which to go, since the child is not, except in the rarest instances, brought to the physician or the psychologist in the very early stages, while the neurosis can be looked upon as incipient. Clearly, if a child of two or three years is seen by ordinary, unspecialized parents to be even a little abnormal, then it is ill indeed. The psychologist, it is true, can make his opportunities of watching ordinary infants and young children; and since, very fortunately, there have been a few parents who have brought their "normal" children for observation or analysis on purely prophylactic grounds, the experienced observer has learnt to read the signs to some extent. It needs, however, a very sensitive perception to recognize the neurotic child in the earliest stages. The inherent difficulties are clearly far greater than in the case of the grown-up, since many things that would mark serious illness in the case of the adult are entirely normal in the young child. It is, for instance, quite normal for the young infant to cry and shout angrily when he cannot get what he wants, to fear the unknown, to empty his bladder and bowels when it pleases him, to depend helplessly upon his mother's love and care. These are the characters of the instinctual life of infancy, and are found in every child, whether or not he becomes neurotic. The problem for us is to know how to distinguish at this early age between, for example, neurotic anxiety and the fear normal to infancy; or, again, between neurotic defiance, hiding deep anxiety, and healthy self-assertion. To know in general that it is a matter of how much and at what age, or of the appropriateness, intensity and fixity of emotion, is one thing; to be able to read the situation precisely in any given case, is another. In the highly intensive and sustained observation afforded by the actual analysis of a child, the diagnosis may be clear enough; but apart from this, and from the cultivated perceptions which such experience brings, I suggest that the reading of the less obvious and dramatic signs of ordinary life is far from easy. Clearly there will always be a general tendency to overlook the earliest indications and to under-estimate their seriousness.

But let us go on to another difficulty, one of perhaps even wider practical import; and that is, that many of the ways of behaviour in a very young child which would at once suggest the possibility or even the certainty of neurosis to the more experienced observer are actually welcomed by the parent and educator as signs of moral development, or chuckled over as evidences of childish quaintness and precocity. A pleasing docility, the absence of open defiance and hostility, particular tidiness, a precise care in folding and arranging the clothes at bed-time, careful effort not to spill water when drinking or washing, anxious dislike of soiled hands or mouth or clothing, solicitude for the return and safety of the mother or the younger child, meticulous kindness and sensitive dislike of cruelty to other children or pet animals, ritual attention to the saying of prayers, frequent endearments and shows of affection, waiting always until one is spoken to before speaking, the offering of gifts to older and stronger children, an ardent desire to be good or clever, an intense ambition not to have to be helped, docility to punishment, drawing-room politeness, the quiet voice and controlled movements—most of these things either please or amuse the parent. Yet any one of them, and particularly several of them found together, may be and often are effects of a deep neurotic guilt and anxiety. The text-books have, of course, long been telling the educator that he must beware of "excessively" good behaviour; the parent who has read anything at all about recent psychology has heard of reaction-formations, and so on. But how is anyone, other than a pure psychologist, and one trained in the study of the neuroses, to know when goodness begins to be excessive, to notice in time that the child is adapting himself only too dangerously well to his "life-task", and the demands of adult values? Above all, how is a parent or educator, whose job is to bring about that very adaptation, to be aware of the deep suffering which may be hidden behind the fair exterior of the good child?

Let me describe a few examples. Among a group of little children which I have recently had the opportunity of observing, under special research conditions, was a charming boy of four years of age, an only child, of not too robust physical health. As was not very surprising, he was at first shy and timid, on being plunged into the group of ten or twelve very vigorous and lively boys running and shouting freely, and sat very quietly watching. Soon, however, he found his feet, and ran and shouted freely with the others, showing, as time went on, increasing initiative and enterprise. He was essentially a good and tractable child, never showing hostility or defiance. There was no trace of priggishness about him, however, and he was very far from being *the* "good child" of the caricature. He was, in fact, distinguished by a robust and delightful sense of humour—he would play at being defiant with the most attractive roguish laughter. Laughter was, indeed, at this stage, the main outlet for his anxieties. For example, he invented a humorous game when using clay, which he very much enjoyed. He pretended that his thumb-nail was coming off, putting a piece of clay on his thumb, and pulling it off, with hearty and infectious laughter. He had, however, before coming to school, shown two symptoms of neurotic anxiety—

occasional frightening dreams which woke him up, and nail-biting. Apart from the nail-biting, his governess had no difficulty in keeping him up to her strict standards of behaviour, and, at home as at school, he was a pleasant and amenable child. After a time, under the freer conditions of the group, his nail-biting almost disappeared, never occurring in school—where, indeed, he now stood out among the other children as an unusually well-adapted child, with a free and vigorous mental life, and great aptitude for happy and constructive play. Yet after a year of apparently most satisfactory intellectual and emotional development, a well-marked neurosis rather suddenly appeared in the shape of constant and severe stammering, and distressing attacks of overt anxiety if he accidentally broke anything, whether his own or another's. He broke a plate at school, for instance, and was overcome by a terrible storm of anxious weeping which no words of comfort could help; and on slightly damaging his own gramophone, refused to touch or look at it again. Fortunately in this case the parents were informed people, and arranged for an analysis. This revealed a deep and severe neurosis, successfully hidden under this fair façade of charm and adaptability, and precipitated by the very freedom on which he had seemed to thrive so gratifyingly. In other words, he had been a good child because his need for punishment for his unconscious libidinal wishes was so great; and when he did not get the censure and strict demands for which he craved, the pressure of the underlying neurosis broke out in unmistakable symptoms. His analyst confirms my impression that any situation of great choice or responsibility in later life, or any circumstances in which free gratification of desire became possible, would have been likely to precipitate the neurosis in this way.

Take another case. A boy of three and a half urinates in his trousers in circumstances which would lead *us* to make every excuse for him, and is overcome by the most heart-rending shame and bitter distress, a shame the intensity of which would again spell neurosis to the experienced student. Yet how difficult for the ordinary parent to see that it is not so much the fact of the "accident" in these circumstances which needs his attention, as the distress which follows it! How can he do other than feel pleased that the child is ashamed of himself?

Another boy of three falls down and hurts his knee; after brief tears, no one being close at hand, he is heard to say reflectively,

"Why should I cry?"   The father reports this with pride and
pleasure, feeling it to be commendable good sense and a delightful
precocity.   But a more skilled observer would see in such a reaction
at this age a too great detachment that hinted not merely at a
high intelligence but also at an overwhelmingly powerful super-
ego.   The same child at five and a half and six years of age showed
periods of unusually successful social adjustment, charm, and
deep affection, alternating with phases of marked querulousness
of an oral type, and inability to bear thwarting, the whole pattern
being woven on a deep underlying melancholy.   And the detachment persisted, with a surprising self-knowledge and self-criticism.
At five and a quarter years, the boy was staying away from home,
and showed a continual and unsatisfiable hunger.   After he had
asked for apples over and over again, someone said to him
laughingly, "You are very hungry, Hugh!"   "Yes," he replied,
"I don't like this house, and that's why I'm always hungry."   Or,
in our words, his being sent away from home to a strange house,
away from the warm and comforting presence of his mother,
re-awakened the earliest deprivation of all, the loss of the nipple
and the resulting oral dissatisfactions.   His penetrating remark
revealed the strength of the oral fixation, and the·extent to which
later experiences would be assimilated to its absolute pattern,
with consequent difficulties in the acceptance of loss.   Out of the
mouth of this babe and suckling came forth wisdom indeed.   And
at six, on having Hiawatha read to him, he asked, "Why was
Hiawatha's father an unkind man?"   Presently supplying his own
answer—"I expect he was unkind because he didn't like himself;
because he didn't like himself, he didn't like other people!"
Again the parents quote his remarks as interesting and delightful
evidences of his high intelligence—as indeed they are; but of
such a kind as to make any student of the individual history of
neurosis watch his development with some anxiety.   This pattern
has persisted to adult life—a rare adaptability and consideration
for others, deep and abiding affections, and devotion to duty,
strong reparative traits of character, but with recurrent moods of
marked self-distrust and depression.

Another type of behaviour in the pre-school child which
naturally delights most parents, but which some of us would
watch very closely as a possible hint of the inner tension which may
later on issue in positive neurosis, is the intense desire to model
himself upon the parent which leads to precocious learning to

read and write. One would at any rate attach importance to this if it were accompanied by any inhibition of pleasure in play and in the expression of fantasy. Again I have definite cases in mind. A boy of barely five, for example, who cannot be persuaded to try modelling in clay because it makes his hands dirty, but who can already read and write up to the normal level of a school child of seven—we are not altogether surprised to find presently that he cannot play happily with a group of children, but must needs torment them into turning on him and making him take a whining refuge with a grown-up, whose hands he clings to convulsively, and only leaves in order to make a furtive attack on the others again, returning at once with a cry of masochistic terror to the protecting adult. The parents are angry when he cries instead of defending himself, and naturally disapprove of his sly attacks on others, treating these things, of course, by moral exhortations; but the precocious reading and writing, and dislike of getting his hands dirty are welcomed and admired. Yet these latter are part of the same psychological picture, and to be also regarded as neurotic symptoms. Sometimes, indeed, the precocity of intellectual development and intense intellectual ambition are the only positive indications of a neurotic diathesis, although they are more safely to be looked upon as such when set amidst a general inhibition of play and fantasy. The child of four and five years who looks on with a bored expression while others romp about pretending to be engines and trains (with his parents again pleased that he is beyond such infantile games); the girl who will not have a birthday party when she is five "because grown-ups don't", and who at two years of age insisted on trying to do everything in the way of climbing or jumping that children several years older were doing, crying out with urgent and shrill anxiety if one went near her—"Don't hold me, don't hold me!" These are spiritual ambitions which I should again watch with some misgivings.

One knows, in all these cases, from the details of analysis that the intense ambition involved points to the severest type of super-ego; and the fact that it has taken a direction which is, on the surface, socially desirable and consonant with adaptation to reality does not compensate for its intensity and despotism. One knows, further, that such intensity indicates that the desire for knowledge and intellectual power is still too strongly libidinised, and itself but a mode of flight from unconscious libidinal wishes, and is therefore liable, at any time of real stress, to suffer from the inroads of guilt. And such a theoretical forecast is amply confirmed from the observation and analysis of adults. Such over-ambitious persons are amongst those who, at the best, are liable in times of severe stress and crisis to attacks of insomnia and depression leading to a "breakdown" which defeats their ends and renders their abilities nugatory.

These, then, are some of the difficulties in the way of the parents' recognition of the earliest signs of neurosis in the pre-school child. Such signs tend to be overlooked either because, on the one hand, they seem to belong to the normal instinctual characteristics of the young child, or because, on the other, they masquerade as welcome signs of growing intelligence and moral development. One might in passing add the further difficulty that the majority of parents would far rather put the trouble down to moral lapses and original sin, even in the case of quite severe neurosis, than admit that a child is in any degree emotionally disturbed—or, as some parents put it—*"mental"*. This springs, of course, from the universal and deep anxiety which makes all ordinary people regard mental disturbance with horror. Like the other difficulties mentioned, it is of importance because, from the nature of the case, the question of the early diagnosis of the neurotic child is necessarily so much in the hands of the parent. Unless and until such time as we have found some way of conveying to the parent and educator the refinements of our own perception of the earliest symptoms of neurosis, our work can hardly be in fact prophylactic.

I have emphasized these difficulties, however, not only because they are relevant to early diagnosis in any particular child, but also because they bear so intimately upon the question of etiology, and, therefore, of practical conclusions. We now know a good deal about the inner conditions of neurosis, and we know something about the external factors. The No Man's Land of comparative ignorance is the exact relation between the inner and outer factors ("between the fixations and the way and the time at which those fixations become connected with experiences," as Mrs. Klein has put it). It might, I think, be said that some of those psychologists who have at this date most confidence in offering prophylactic advice to the educator are the ones who lay most weight upon the external precipitating factors. They emphasize either the simple traumatic theory, in which a shock of some kind is held responsible for the neurosis—an attack by an animal, a threat of castration, a seduction, an actual viewing of parental coitus, the infant's being half-suffocated by the large pendulous breast of a careless mother, and so on; or the same theory in a more veiled form, in which the general behaviour and characteristics of the parents, their day-to-day words and moods and actions, are held to be the effective cause. It is, of course, true that these external factors are the only ones we can alter, or most readily alter; and optimism naturally turns its gaze in their direction. Yet until we have more understanding of the precise interplay of inner fixation and actual experience, where the crux lies, optimism must needs be curbed. And for this understanding, we need the most precise and intensive knowledge of both inner tendency and outer circumstance. It seems to me that it may be theoretically very misleading to base any possible principles of prophylaxis on merely *extensive* data, on a surface comparison of cases showing well-developed symptoms; and that comparative data of an intensive kind, based upon the earliest possible diagnosis, and upon the detailed observation afforded by actual analysis, are indispensable. For these reasons I have ventured to emphasize, as a first consideration, the practical difficulties in the way of early diagnosis.

II

PRIVATION AND GUILT[1]

(1929)

I

IN his paper on "The Origin and Structure of the Super-Ego,"[2] in 1926, Ernest Jones prefaced his discussion of some of the problems arising out of this topic with the remark that "there is every reason to think that the concept of the super-ego is a nodal point where we may expect all the obscure problems of the Œdipus complex and narcissism on the one hand, and hate and sadism on the other, to meet". Since that date, contributions towards the further elucidation of these issues have been made by Freud and others, and our knowledge of the structure and modes of functioning of the super-ego, in the neuroses, psychoses and normal character, has been greatly amplified.

On the other hand, the results of Melanie Klein's direct researches into the minds of very young children, whilst underlining the theoretical value of the concept of the super-ego, and deepening our sense of its enormous dynamic power, have nevertheless increased certain of the theoretical difficulties attaching to the first modes of statement of its origin, of its relation to the Œdipus complex, and the developmental phases of the libido. To my mind, the most illuminating suggestion which has yet been offered on these tangled issues is that made by Jones (elaborating a hint of Freud's), when he says that *privation is equivalent to frustration*[3]. He further remarks, " . . . guilt, and with it the super-ego, is as it were artificially built up for the purpose of protecting the child from the stress of privation, i.e. of ungratified libido, and so warding off the dread of aphanisis that always goes with this; it does so, of course, by damping down the wishes that are not destined to be gratified. I even think that the external disapproval, to which the whole of this process used to be ascribed,

---

[1] *International Journal of Psycho-Analysis*, Vol. X, Pts. 2 and 3. 1929.
[2] *I.J.P.A.*, Vol. VII, pp. 303 *et seq.*
[3] "The Early Development of Female Sexuality," *I.J.P.A.* Vol., VIII, p. 463,

is largely an affair of exploitation on the child's part; that is to say, non-gratification primarily means danger, and the child projects this into the outer world, as it does with all internal dangers, and then makes use of any disapproval that comes to meet it there (*moralisches Entgegenkommen*) to signalize the danger and to help it in constructing a barrier against this".

My desire in this paper is to set out (*a*) some of the difficulties which appear to arise when the earlier formulas for the origin of the super-ego are set against the facts of mental history discovered directly by Melanie Klein's technique; and (*b*) to suggest how this view of Ernest Jones', together with his concept of *aphanisis*, appear to resolve these difficulties.

To state the difficulties first:

After reading a series of the earlier accounts of the genesis of the super-ego, one is left with the impression that a certain time-relation between this and the Œdipus complex was conceived to hold. Freud's classic phrase that the super-ego is "the heir of the Œdipus complex" hints strongly that the former is held to appear as and when the latter dies out; and this view is also emphasized in both the title and the substance of "The Passing of the Œdipus Complex".[1] It comes into explicit expression in the following: "I have no doubt that the temporal and causal relations described between the Œdipus complex, sexual intimidation (the threat of castration), formation of the super-ego and advent of the latency period, are of a typical kind".

This, then, was the general point of view, previous to Klein's work, with regard to the time and mode of onset of the super-ego, viz. that it belonged essentially to the phallic stage of libidinal development, was the outcome of the frustration and anxieties experienced by the child in his object-relationships at that level, and signalized the passing of the Œdipus complex and the beginning of the latency period.

Now this way of stating the history of the super-ego has clearly to be modified in order to fit the fuller facts offered by Melanie Klein as the outcome of her direct investigations of very young children.

There are two main points to be considered here. (1) Both in

---

[1] *Collected Papers*, Vol. II, p. 269. Freud then goes on to reserve some doubts as to the part played by the dread of castration, doubts aroused by Rank's work on the birth trauma; and to which he returns in *Hemmung, Symptom und Angst*, 1926. This latter is obviously also closely relevant to the issues I am raising, and the development of Freud's views therein clearly coincides in direction with Jones' contribution.

"The Psychological Principles of Infant Analysis",[1] and "The Early Stages of the Œdipus Conflict",[2] Melanie Klein develops her conclusion that "the Œdipus complex comes into operation earlier than is usually supposed", and that "the very onset of the Œdipus wishes . . . already becomes associated with incipient dread of castration and feelings of guilt". She thinks it is no longer possible to hold that the guilt found to be linked up, in the analysis of adults, with the pregenital impulses is "of subsequent growth, displaced back on to these tendencies, though not originally associated with them". Going beyond the hints given by Ferenczi and Abraham in this connection, she says, "My findings lead rather further. They show that the sense of guilt associated with pregenital fixation is already the direct effect of the Œdipus conflict. And this seems to account satisfactorily for the genesis of such feelings, for we know the sense of guilt to be simply a result of the introjection (already accomplished, or, as I would add, *in process of being accomplished*),[3] of the Œdipus love-objects".

The formation of the super-ego, thus, so far from being a single psychic act, or even a process which can be placed mainly within a single phase of development, the phallic, is seen to be interwoven with all developmental phases, to have its deepest roots in oral experiences, and to run on continuously throughout all the emotional vicissitudes of the child, from the breast to the latency period.

(2) The second point, closely connected with the first, and made very clear by Klein, is that the parents "introjected"[4] are not the *real* parents, with their real characteristics, but *the parents as apprehended by the child through the medium of his own active psychology.* This is put most clearly in her contribution to the "Symposium on Child Analysis", p. 356.[5] "For these external objects (i.e. the parents) are certainly not identical with the already developed super-ego of the child, even though they have at one time contributed to its development. It is only thus that we can explain the astonishing fact that in children of three, four and five years

---

[1] *I.J.P.A.*, Vol. VIII, Pt. 1.
[2] Ibid.. Vol. IX, Pt. 2.
[3] Present writer's italics.
[4] "The authority of the father or the parents is introjected into the ego, and there forms the kernel of the super-ego, which takes its severity from the father, perpetuates his prohibition against incest, and so ensures the ego against a recurrence of the libidinal object-cathexis." "The Passing of the Œdipus Complex."
[5] *I.J.P.A.*, Vol. VIII, Pt. 3.

old we encounter a super-ego of a severity which is often in the sharpest contradiction to the real love-objects, the parents." Or, again, "the connection between the formation of the super-ego and the pregenital phases of development is very important from two points of view. On the one hand, the sense of guilt attaches itself to the oral- and anal-sadistic phases, which as yet predominate; and, on the other, the super-ego comes into being while these phases are in the ascendant, which accounts for its sadistic severity." The structure of the super-ego is thus "built up of identifications dating from very different periods and strata in the mental life".

Now these views, whilst they make some aspects of the super-ego at once more intelligible—as, for instance, its fantastic severity, and its independence of the real character of the parents—nevertheless raise certain further theoretical difficulties. It is, for example, not easy to see at first sight how and why guilt, as distinct from primary anxiety, should arise at the oral stage—since guilt would seem to imply some definite measure of distinction between the self and the not-self, and would seem to rest upon some degree of object-relationship, which as yet must be only rudimentary. The picture of ego-modifications as the result of abandoned object-cathexes, in the phallic or later genital phases, is quite clear. "When the ego assumes the features of the object, it forces itself, so to speak, upon the id as a love-object, and tries to make good the loss of that object by saying, 'Look, I am so like the object, you can as well love me'."[1] But in what ways can this be seen to hold of the relatively undifferentiated "object" and "me" in the earlier phases?

Obviously, the process of "introjection" in these earlier phases must be different in some important sense from that occurring after there has been true object-relationship. Nor, perhaps, is this difference fully covered by pointing out that in these early stages the object is but a *part*-object—the nipple, the mother's bowel-contents, long before the mother. That the "me" predominates over the "not-me" is made clear because, as Klein shows, the child apprehends the parents only as it apprehends itself, and in terms of its own impulses. It is not the *parents* who are "introjected", but a distorted imago, the psychic contents of which are derived rather, perhaps, from *projection*. The mechanism of introjection yields the form, the externality of the super-ego

[1] Freud, *The Ego and the Id*, p. 37.

in relation to the id; but it is projection which determines its concrete mode of operation (cutting, biting, destroying, etc.). Or, to put it differently, it is very truly a part of the child's own psyche which is differentiated to act as if it were external to the id impulses. One suspects that Freud's "primary identification"[1] may perhaps play a greater part in the total drama than was originally thought.

Again, in what sense or senses can we understand the dictum that "anxiety of conscience is internalized castration anxiety", at these early stages? This is clear and understandable for the phallic phase—but not so easily to be read as one runs for the anal and oral, in spite of the already familiar notions of the loss of the nipple and bowel-contents.

These and other difficulties of clear statement crowd upon one. What follows is a partial and very tentative attempt to get round them. I do not propose to take them one by one, but to try to re-phrase the problem of the early onset of guilt along the lines of Jones' view that "privation is equivalent to frustration". I do so in the hope that my fragmentary remarks may provoke others to clarify these problems further.

2

From the moment when the travail of the mother begins, experience for the child is a series of disturbances of equilibrium, of moments of increase in tension, and more or less successful discharge of tension. The part played by the first and severest of these disturbances, birth itself, is now (since *Hemmung, Symptom und Angst*) clear in many respects. Birth, because of the suddenness and intensity of the stimuli the child then suffers, and his psychic helplessness in face of these, arouses the first and greatest anxiety-state. This acute birth helplessness is the prototype of all later anxieties, the further occasions being probably a milder re-activation of this original reaction.

Now here we may also make use of an interesting set of facts gained from recent direct studies of infant behaviour. The

---

[1] "At the very beginning, in the primitive oral phase of the individual's existence, object-cathexis and identification are hardly to be distinguished from each other"; *The Ego and the Id*, p. 35.

"This, the first and most important identification of all, is apparently not in the first instance the consequence or outcome of an object-cathexis; it is a direct and immediate identification, and takes place earlier than any object-cathexis," p. 39.

experimental studies by Watson of the innate responses of the infant in the earliest days following birth yield data which fit in well with Freud's view. There are two kinds of external stimuli which call out the fear-reaction in the earliest days— sudden loss of support, and a sudden loud noise. (These may both be called real dangers, and may be contrasted with the phobias appearing later, the earliest true phobias instanced by Freud, viz. being alone, being in the dark, being with strangers; these are reactions to *the absence of the loved person*, and may already be looked upon as neurotic.)

A sudden loud noise reduces the child to the state of psychic shock and helplessness which is anxiety, since he cannot move away from or shut out the too intense stimulus, as he can shut out, for example, too intense a light, by closing his eyes and turning away his head. He has no ear-lids to close!

Sudden loss of support, if the child is dropped or his blanket twitched when he is falling to sleep, is in the same way a real danger, and one that will from the nature of the case readily re-animate the birth anxiety. This will have in it, however, not only the element of real danger, but the seeds of the later fear of *loss of object*—since support in the mother's arms must itself be libidinally toned, meaning love as well as safety.

It is illuminating here to contrast for a moment the theoretical use which Watson makes of the facts he so carefully gathers, with the insight of Freud. On Watson's view, all *later* phobias are derived from these two by environmental "conditioning". Because they (the fears of the dark, of strangers, of particular animals, etc.) appear later, he assumes this to mean that they are therefore environmentally, rather than psychically, conditioned. For him, the instance of the later fear—the dark or the animal—is a sign, a condition, of the earlier instance, built up into one pattern with it by reflex association.

For Freud, also, these particular later phobias are secondary phenomena—signs and conditions; but of tensions arising from *inner* stimuli. The anxiety is real, no less than in well-grounded fears of real outer dangers; but the danger apprehended is the state of psychic helplessness as the result of overwhelming *inner* tension which cannot be adequately discharged; and which is thus reacted to *as if it were an external danger*.

And these inner stimuli in the earliest days are the component sexual impulses at the oral and anal levels of sexual development—

the libidinal element in sucking and biting, in the passing of fæces or their accumulation within the bowel; and the first object-relationships connected with these erogenous zones. The phantasies made plain in the later play of children, as well as in the psychoses and neuroses of adults, show that these object-relationships take the form of the desire, first, to incorporate the object (= mother's nipple), then to bite and destroy it; and later to find out and appropriate the contents of her body (bowel-womb); and to destroy rivals (father or other children) who might stand in the way of satisfaction. Presently, when the phallic phase sets in, the desire is to see and possess the genital of the loved person; and, again, to remove and destroy all rivals.

(Melanie Klein insists, and it helps our difficulties to keep in mind, that these phases in libidinal development overlap and merge into each other very intimately throughout the early years. In other words, even when the child has progressed to the more developed object-relationship of the phallic level, he is bound to be yet so insecurely planted there that his phallic impulses and phantasies will be deeply infused with the characteristics belonging to the pregenital zones and pregenital impulses.)

Two questions at once arise: (1) How and why should these early libidinal trends awake anxiety? And (2) at what age do they begin to do so?

To take the second first. No precise time can be indicated from the available evidence. But it will be *at such time as some measure of true object-relationship has developed*, even though the object be mainly one apprehended in terms of oral experience. That is to say, the nipple-breast-mother will then (at whatever point in the series nipple-breast-mother this may happen) be already well distinguished as *something not-me*, which the *me* wants, has, loses, wants again and has again, and so on—in a series of changes which come and go within the field of the *me*, but which are outside its control. It probably can only happen at a time when, although the nipple-breast remains the important part of the mother, the core of her meaning, she is something well beyond this in richness and articulation of perceptual content. When, in other words, the exteroceptors of the child are sufficiently educated and synthesized, and the memory-traces of the ego sufficiently developed, as to make the perception of a *person* (in some terms) possible (this being, in its turn, dependent upon the loosening of the libido from its primary narcissistic investment); and yet, at such a time when there is still a huge element of *primary identifica-tion* involved in this perception—of filling out the content of the perception with the *me's* own visceral and kinæsthetic ex-periences, and id impulses.

The evidence seems to suggest any time within the second half of the first year, varying with the child, and possibly with cir-cumstance (such as the age of weaning, the oversight or hearing of parental coitus, etc. But much remains to be known here). Undoubtedly, well before the end of the first year with some children, and during the early part of the second year with others, direct observation will show developed sufficient sense of persons and of relationship to persons as to make possible manifestations of jealousy and of rage aroused by jealousy; of a direct response of fear to frowns and angry looks on the faces of loved people; and of anxieties other than those called out by intense or sudden outer stimuli.

Now to return to the first question. Until the suggestion made by Jones, already referred to, and the remarks leading in the same direction by Joan Riviere, in her paper in the "Symposium on Child Analysis",[1] the tendency was to look upon the experience of weaning, and the real behaviour of the parents in ordering the training in cleanliness, as determining causes of guilt. Now, however, we should be more inclined to regard them simply as occasions.

At first sight there is little theoretical difficulty about the part played by training in cleanliness. One knows that this *is* usually done in such a way as deliberately to foster the feeling of re-sponsibility in the child. The long-continued active pressure brought to bear upon him, urging to the control of the sphincters, no matter how pleasantly and patiently done, is clearly of the same psychological order as his own feeling of guilt. The parents *do* set conditions to the continuance of their love; there is real frustration, as distinct from privation. (Further reflection suggests, it is true, that even here the situation is more com-plicated than this; the severity of the guilt aroused, for example, is too great to be explained away by this real situation.)

Very few parents, however, make a moral affair of weaning. It is far more usually a simple matter-of-fact change, and done with care and sympathy. How then should it give rise to guilt in the child? Melanie Klein's term is that the anal and oral

[1] *I.J.P.A.*, Vol. VIII, p. 370.

frustrations "release" the Œdipus tendencies; and with them, guilt.

Is it possible to articulate more fully the steps which lead from oral privation to guilt and the super-ego?

It is, in the first place, obvious that a great heaping-up of oral libido, of the impulses which have hitherto enjoyed some measure of real satisfaction, but which are now thwarted, will occur; and will lead to a sense of unbearable tension and psychic helplessness. Rage and hate impulses will, as a result, greatly augment the sadistic element in the love of the nipple-breast-mother, which itself is commonly one of the conditions of the weaning. There will be a considerable heightening of the awareness of *things-not-me*, and thus of object-relationships. These will be primarily objects which are interfering, denying and therefore hostile, *things-which-thwart-me*, and which *me* would destroy if it could; but, nevertheless, there will be this heightening of object-sense, and of the search for an object on which to discharge the heaped-up libido. *An object which cannot yet be found.* For, quite apart from the will and pleasure of the parents, the nature of the oral-sadistic impulses is such that they cannot really be satisfied—neither the love nor the hate. The child wants not only to bite the nipple—as he will do if allowed; but to destroy all thwarting objects and rival persons; and even the loved mother, by way of love. That is what he is at this stage—a creature who loves and hates *with his mouth and teeth;* and can no other.

Underlying the real moral element in the anal training, moreover, are the same fundamental privations. Apprehending, loving and hating in terms of his bowel experiences, the child desires and phantasies the fulfilment of desires which never can be realized in fact. He "desires to get possession of the mother's fæces, by penetrating into her body, cutting it to pieces, devouring it and destroying it".[1] And along with this sadistic and possessive love of his mother, itself permeated with the hatred aroused by her oral interferences, goes his hate and dread of his father. (The first onset of the genital impulses takes place under the ægis of this sadistic phase; hence the strength and spontaneity of the castration fears.)

There are two further considerations which strengthen these hints that the privation set up by weaning may but serve to augment and give point to the privations inherent in the oral

[1] "The Early Stages of the Œdipus Conflict," p. 170.

and anal libidinal situations. In the first place, the pregenital zones appear to be relatively segmental and isolated in their functioning, and to be incapable of the full discharge of the libidinal tension of the whole body, as may occur with the genital orgasm under favourable psychological conditions. And secondly, all demands at these levels are of too timeless, ungraded and absolute a nature to find complete satisfaction in a real world limited by time and space conditions.

One therefore sees the trauma of weaning as perhaps but applying the match to a fire of already prepared dissatisfaction, inherent in the libidinal situation at this stage. And the later anal privations add fuel to this fire.

This intolerable tension would reduce the weak and young ego to a state of psychic helplessness approximating to that of birth itself, were it not dealt with somehow. And it is dealt with by projecting the danger to the ego into the outside world, as external frustration. From there it later returns, like the thrown boomerang, into the psyche, as guilt and the super-ego—now charged with the power and authority of the external, thwarting, world.

This latest stage of guilt must, however, be built upon the first stage of "primary identification", and what in all likelihood go along with it, the earlier among Ferenczi's "stages in the development of the sense of reality".

We can thus perhaps decipher five main stages in the whole process. The first has itself three main aspects: (a) primary auto-erotism, antedating all object-cathexes; (b) an almost complete "omnipotence"—omnipotence conditioned by subjective changes, phantasies, gestures, cries, and the like. The exteroceptors and musculature are not yet developed enough to make perception of things and persons possible; (c) primary identification, in which the outer world (= persons) is drawn into the circle of the psyche. At this stage, the *me* is much more solid and continuous than the sporadic incursions of the *not-me*. These are (at first) isolated, without relations, and therefore without meaning. The events in the *me* must be much more closely linked up and continuous, and the first effect of the *not-me* shocks must be simply to throw the *me* into high relief. The former will be laid hold of in terms of the latter, and assimilated to it. Hence there must be already a tendency on the part of the *me* to assume responsibility for events in so far as they are pleasurable, to refer intrusions of the external to preceding internal changes. For only so can they be (illusorily) controlled before there is perceptual discrimination of specific cause and effect.

In the characteristic moments of this stage "the ego-subject coincides with what is pleasurable and the outside world with what is indifferent (or even painful as being a source of stimulation)".[1] External events which bring discomfort are turned away from—as it were, closed over by the flow of narcissistic libido.

One can perhaps see this element reflected even in certain later phases. For example, one motive in the much later identification of the girl with the father (when this occurs) may be the desire for control of the conditions of pleasure. If the penis (= nipple) is her own (part of the *me*), then she can enjoy it as and when she wishes, free from the to-her-merely-arbitrary will of others. This, of course, is partly built upon the object-directed anal desire for mastery, and oral desire for possession, as well as the true Œdipus relation; but still further below the identification may be this reference of all sources of pleasure to *me* as sufficient cause.

This first stage will pass over continuously and imperceptibly into the second—as presently, the second into the third.

The second stage is that of the earliest object-cathexes, and rudimentary object-relationships.

The possibility of object-relationships has two concurrent and inter-related aspects: (1) the growing strength of the ego, which comes to have less need of narcissistic libido; and (2) the increase in the variety, connectedness and continuity of external stimuli. It may be presumed that outer events come to be tolerated in attention (not turned away from altogether, as in the primary narcissistic stage) only as they become linked up with an end-state of pleasure, and thus, conditions of satisfaction. External perceptions thus come to have enough relatedness to be referred to external conditions, and, to a greater or less extent, distinguished from internal happenings. These external events must, of course, themselves be apprehended at first as personal agencies, in terms of the internal causal series. Just as in the first stage the *me* assimilates external events in order to control them, so, in this second stage, it does so (in form) in order to *understand* and so control them, by acting on them. It feels them to be outside itself, but like itself.

When this perceptual ordering of the external world in terms of

[1] Freud, "Instincts and Their Vicissitudes", *Collected Papers*, Vol. IV, p. 78.

personal agency, together with the appropriate object-cathexes, has been reached, the stage is set for the reference of internal libidinal tension in its turn to external danger. This is the time when "the ego thrusts forth upon the external world whatever within itself gives rise to pain";[1] when *privation becomes equivalent to frustration.* "I haven't got what I want" becomes "You deny me". This gap is crossed on the slender real bridge of the actual with-holding of the pleasures of the breast by the mother.

"I am afraid of my helplessness before my own sadistic desires" is thus turned into "I fear your cruel thwarting"; and this is further developed into "You thwart me *because* I wish to possess and destroy you". "You took it from me *because* I wanted to bite." It is this *because* which acts as the needed barrier to the uprush of libido. And the thwarting agencies (as Klein makes so clear and as we have seen must inevitably be so) are given all the intemperateness and ruthlessness of the child's own pent-up impulses. What is feared, as Jones has shown, is retaliatory injury to the body involving total extinction of pleasure. It is this dread of *aphanisis* which is in due course specified and local-ized as castration-fear; and which is in the third stage internalized again in its turn.

The earliest components of guilt thus belong to the least diffe-rentiated and graded levels of experience. From the fact that the first and most powerful object-cathexes occur here, guilt draws its all-or-none-ness and automaticity. This it is which causes the later "conscience" to remain a "categorical imperative" in its mode of operation, its not-to-be-questioned-ness, even when its specific content and incidence in the objective world is infused with discriminated reality.

It would seem to be on this background of the sense of being thwarted by the punishing mother for sadistic desires towards her that the more complicated cross-relationships of the Œdipus situation are embroidered. Mrs. Klein suggests that the oral (and anal) frustrations "release the Œdipus tendencies"; and perhaps, with them, the incipient genital phase.

And so we come to the third stage, when we pass from the sense of frustration to guilt proper; when the love-objects are "intro-jected", and the castration-anxiety proper is internalized.

If we were to logicize this process of internalization, the steps might run something like this:

[1] "Instincts and Their Vicissitudes."

(*a*) "You thwart me because I wish to possess and/or destroy you."

(*b*) "If I do not wish to possess and/or destroy you, you will love (= not hate) me."

(*c*) "I will thwart myself, because I hate you." (Consciously, "because I love (= do not hate) you".)

(*d*) "I can love myself if I thwart myself."

(*e*) "I love myself if I love (= do not hate) you."

And (*e*) would be the logic of the normal conscience, on the genital level; (*c*) that of the obsessional.

Things do not, of course, happen so simply. At every step there is in fact the most complex shuttle-like back and forth movement between the internal and the external—just as there is in later history between the super-ego and the id.

Of the general dynamic and economic functions of this internalization there is no need to speak here. One point may be made, viz. that it makes for the development of the real ego and for knowledge and control of the external world—both by withdrawing the stress of control of the id from the ego, and by freeing external events from their over-investment with libidinal values.

I have, in this very fragmentary and tentative paper, been primarily interested in the second stage of the genesis of guilt, because it is there that (to my mind) the greater obscurities still remain. One conclusion is reinforced by the facts and considerations here dealt with, viz. the inevitability of guilt in the human mind. It arises from the developmental processes themselves, in the child, and not from his accidental circumstances or faulty education. It is not to be explained (away) by false theologies; but they by it.

III

REBELLIOUS AND DEFIANT CHILDREN[1]

(1934)

THIS subject concerns everyone, since all children at one time or another and in one way or another are rebellious and defiant. Some children are markedly so throughout the whole of their development; it becomes their characteristic way of responding to all adults and authorities. They show defiance and hate more continuously, more intensely, or with less obvious provocation than most others, and the mode of behaviour may become a settled response in adult life. The extreme cases are delinquent children and habitual adult criminals.

I am concerned to-night mainly with *open* rebellion. Many a violent revolution goes on behind a docile front, and never shows itself openly. The too-good child is usually welcome at home and easily overlooked in school, whatever his age. He may, however, be in a more serious psychological state than the frankly defiant child, and his way of dealing with his feelings may ultimately lead to severe mental illness. We have more reason to be troubled about him than about the rebels, except in very marked cases.

EXAMPLES AND AGE DIFFERENCES

Rebelliousness and defiance are, however, normally characteristic of certain periods of development in healthy children. E.g. (*a*) in the second and third years: the study of temper tantrums, which appear as extreme expressions of defiance, shows that there is a high peak on the curve of incidence in the second and third years. (*b*) Again at seven to eight years, when children go through a period of special anxiety which issues in defiance and rebellion. This anxiety is in part at least connected with the second teething.[2] (*c*) In early adolescence, when defiance and rebelliousness are probably shown in their most dramatic

---

[1] A lecture given to a general public audience at the Institute of Psycho-Analysis 1934. Not previously published.
[2] Note (1947). See Gesell: *The Child from Five to Ten.* 1947.

form and are often difficult for parents, teachers and social institutions to cope with.

The types of rebellion shown in early adolescence will be familiar to you all, e.g. arguing and "answering back", staying out late, refusing to go to bed at a reasonable hour, persisting with friends disapproved of by the parents, truancy, wandering, stealing—these instances merging into delinquency proper. One of the main differences between the younger child and the adolescent is that the older boy or girl is able to be defiant in a more effective way than the younger.[1]

Apart from adolescence, it may be interesting to compare the different ways in which children express their defiance at different ages. Here are some examples received from their mothers and nurses, of children under and over five years of age:—

Under Five Years

"She (aged two years, three months) simply hates being dressed in the morning, having her hair brushed and face and hands washed. She fights and kicks and screams and bites."

"Whenever I pick Alan (aged one year, eleven months) up to dress him or undress him, he flings himself back rigid across my lap, not crying or upset at all, but just looking determined. It makes it impossible to dress him and it usually ends up with my losing my temper and giving him a sharp smack, which certainly makes him obey me but which I feel is quite the wrong way to treat him, and yet what else can I do? I have also tried standing him up to dress him, but he simply won't stand up but slides down on to the floor and lies there. You have no idea how maddening this is morning after morning when I am in a hurry!"

"I am quite at sea as to the best way of managing my little boy of two-and-a-half-years. Everything is a struggle. He says 'No' to everything and it is a fight to make him do what I want and not to give in to him. He screams, yells, sits down in the middle of the road. If he does not get his own way he whines and cries, and smacks and pinches those around him. He also bites. He really makes things very unhappy as life is a continual battle."

"My small boy of four has a very strong spirit of contrariness. This is the kind of thing which occurs. When out for a walk he

---

[1] Note (1947). It was found, for example, during the early part of the 1939–44 war, when children were evacuated from the cities to country towns, that whereas the little ones and those of the middle years might be difficult and unhappy, and especially, might wet their beds, some of those of thirteen and fourteen years simply took the law into their own hands and returned home. (See *Cambridge Evacuation Survey*.)

saw on a gate leading to the front of a hotel, IN, and on the next gate, OUT; and remarked, 'It says IN and OUT on these gates. I will go in where it says OUT and out where it says IN.' "

"It is of three-year-old Isabelle I write. Lately she has taken a delight in doing all the things she knows are naughty, such as jumping on the bed (which she helps me to make), playing with things she knows perfectly well she ought not to touch, such as baby's teats, standing on a chair to reach them. She insists on drinking her bath water. In fact her whole day is spent in this way, which is very unhappy for all of us."

Over Five Years

"No matter what you ask J. (aged five years, six months) to do the first thing which comes to his lips is 'No'. Any treat you propose, anything he especially likes offered him at table, produces an instant 'Don't want it'. We always suggest things to him as if we knew he meant to accept and cheerfully, but the answer is always in the negative. We have tried taking no notice of his refusals, but he persists in refusing until we say, 'Oh! very well, you don't want it'. Then he says he does and cries bitterly if the cake or whatever was offered him is removed. If it is then handed to him he will again say he doesn't want it and this may go on several times, when finally it is removed for good. Sometimes when he fears he is really losing it he will give in and accept it sooner."

"V. has developed the most annoying habit of contradicting everything. For instance, when the back door bell rang the other day my mother said, 'There's the milkman!' V. said 'Tisn't', and it was. I tell her to put on a certain coat or pair of shoes and say 'because it's cold' or 'because it's going to rain', and she says 'it *isn't* cold', and so on. When we are out she'll say, 'What's that?' pointing to something we are passing, and when I explain she says, 'Don't be silly, it isn't'. She also contradicts herself."

"Another difficulty with Peter (nearly seven) is that he really does not seem to mind being punished. I have tried all kinds of punishments, sending him to bed, depriving him of sweets, etc. Whipping, I am sure, merely hardens him. He will listen with a heart-rending expression of penitence to a 'good talking-to' whether delivered with anger or merely in sorrowful exhortation, and disappointment! But the *moment* it is over, his tears and distress vanish miraculously, as if they had never been, and he is down again playing with his train upon the floor. If brought to book for obvious disobedience, he will glibly recite what he has done, and what he was told *not* to do, showing that he did not just *forget*, but deliberately disobeyed, knowing he was doing wrong. But he will rarely tell a lie to save himself, and looks one fearlessly in the eyes even when in a serious 'row'."

"My little girl is nearly eight years old. When alone with me, she is most interesting and charming, but when playing with her little brother and sister, or ragging with her Daddy, she seems to delight in deliberately annoying people. Sometimes she comes up to me and says, 'Now I'm going to annoy you', and does all the things she knows I dislike and keeps looking surreptitiously at me to see if it is having the desired effect."

We can thus say that whereas under four to five years, defiance and hatred are mostly shown in fighting, kicking, going rigid and other forms of temper tantrum, in the middle years they appear more typically as indifference, hardness, "turning a deaf ear", contradictoriness and "deliberate" disobedience.

MOTIVES FOR REBELLION AND DEFIANCE

Have these various types of rebellion in different children and at various ages any common elements? Psycho-analytic experience with rebellious and difficult children (and adults), as well as many observations in ordinary life, have shown that the determinants of such behaviour are very complex. There are underlying motives common to all, but also many individual meanings.

Any child will, of course, be made rebellious if the adults behave in a way which cuts across all his normal and healthy impulses of development: e.g. if a child of eighteen months is treated as "naughty" for taking his gloves off in his pram, or one of three years is scolded for wanting to wash his own hands instead of standing quiet and good while his nurse does this for him; if a boy of thirteen or fourteen years is not allowed the slightest choice of action or freedom of speech, but expected always to behave as if he were still a little child, we do not feel surprised to see him rebel. Again, we are all now familiar with the fact that illegitimacy and a broken home contribute heavily to. rebellion against the social order, and may lead to delinquency.

But attitudes of defiance and hatred are not confined to children whose homes are either ununderstanding or seriously bad, that is to say where there are avoidable situations of un-happiness. Circumstances which cannot be helped, such as financial trouble in the family, the birth of a new baby, the illness or death of a loved adult, or merely being the eldest or the youngest child, and all the complex interplay of the tempera-mental characteristics of different children in the same family, things which nobody can be blamed for, may enhance the normal tendency to rebelliousness by setting emotional problems which the particular child does not seem able to solve in any other way than by defiance and hardness.

A common notion about rebellious children of any age is that they are "wilfully naughty", and do not *want* to be "good" or docile or friendly. There is an element of truth in this. There is usually a wish mixed up with other motives, a pleasure in defeating the adults. For instance a little girl has wishes arising from her direct rivalry with her mother, which may be present at a very early age. She may not want mother to have a good child—in the shape of herself or any other child. She wants babies of her own, and as she cannot have them, may prefer to reproach mother with having a bad one, or to get her into trouble with father; or she wants to get the nurse into trouble with the mother. But by itself this notion of mere "wilfulness" is far too simple an explanation. The wish motive has to be recognised as a genuine element in the whole phenomenon, but it is by no means the sole one, as it is so often imagined to be. There is often also a wish to help the mother and to make her children good, as well as to be good oneself, wishes which cannot operate effectively because of deeper and earlier drives and anxieties.

Using the knowledge gained from psycho-analytic work with children and adults, let us look more closely at some of the complex motives entering into acts of defiance and feelings of hatred.

Hatred is in itself as primitive an instinct as love, but it may be used as a *defence* against feelings of love (or more accurately, against all the anxieties which go along with feelings of love) just as in other cases love, docility and charm may be used as a defence against secret hatred.[1] That is one of the things we have

---

[1] Note (1947). See *The Psycho-Analysis of Children*, 1932; and "A Contribution to the Psychogenesis of Manic-Depressive States", *I.J.P.A.*, Vol. XVI. 1935, as well as various later papers, by Melanie Klein; also *Love, Hate and Reparation* by Melanie Klein and Joan Riviere, 1937, in which these matters are far more adequately and fully dealt with.

slowly come to understand—the way in which particular tendencies or feelings may be held on to and over-emphasised in
order to keep at bay others which are more painful, i.e. they
become *defences* against the inner awareness of the more painful
feelings or against impulses felt to be more dangerous.

In characteristically defiant children hate is being used as a
defence against the frustrations and fears connected with love,
i.e. not only against the pain of loss and frustration, but also
against depression and sadness and the fear of damaging the
loved object by greed and possessiveness. The unconscious argument in its simplest form runs: "If you won't love me and give
me all I want, I cannot and won't love you. Indeed I don't love
you, I *hate* you." In the end, however, the child feels that if he
has *only* hatred for his mother, and does not want what she has,
then he is neither frustrated, nor need he be anxious about the
harm his greed and possessiveness may do. Adolescent and
adult patients sometimes openly express the feeling of how much
simpler life would be if one could do nothing but hate. And in the
analytic work, when the earliest love for the mother or the father,
which has been buried under the layers of hatred and defiance,
is brought to light, the pain and suffering of the patient on realis-
ing the depth and extent of this love, and of the complex interplay
of his love and hate, may be extreme. The attitude of "sour
grapes" is an important element in the boy's turning away from
his mother in the latency period, as well as in the defiance of
adolescence and in the girl's tomboyish rebellion of the middle
years. It is a safety device, directed against incestuous sexual
wishes and against feelings of love, grief and despair.

Related to this is the use of hate and defiance as a defence
against the sense of obligation, against the wish or need to repair
and restore what has been damaged, the fear that one has not
enough "good" inside oneself to do so. The child's ego dreads
lest everything good in himself (the good food, the good breast
and the good parents whom he feels he has taken into himself)
may have to be wholly devoted to restoring the damaged objects
and that thus there will be no "good", no pleasure or happiness
left for him; or he fears that in any case there is not enough good
to restore the damaged objects. It thus seems better to deny any
sense of obligation and refuse any effort. There is often a great
dread of the feeling "I *ought* to be good". The efforts which are
called for are imagined as unending and all-exhausting. The little

child often feels this when his mother is ill, or if he hears his parents talk in his presence about money or other acute problems which trouble them; he feels guilty because of what they do for him, and imagines that he ought to be able to do something marvellous to help them. It is hard for him at the same time to wish to help them and to recognise that he is not able.to do so in any effective way, and he may then deny that he wants to help them and turn to the pleasures of hate and destruction instead.

We thus have the use of hate as a defence against unconscious guilt. Instead of feeling "mother is ill because I was naughty and made her so", and being aware of guilt and sorrow about it, as he does in the depths of his heart, the child finds it easier to see mother as "bad" in herself and only fit to be hated. In this way he feels relieved of guilt because he projects upon her the badness in himself. It is not his fault if she seems bad; she is so by nature. She *is* unkind or mean or cruel. This is an extremely common element both in occasional and in more sustained attitudes of hate and defiance. It is resorted to when guilt is too strong to be borne, either for reasons of reality, if very distressing things have actually happened in the child's environment, or because for inner reasons the child has strongly developed phantasies of punishment.

Another use of hatred and defiance is as a defence against the fear of the dangers which spring from gratification, the fear of getting what one wants. This is a fear which arises much more from phantasy than from reality, and is at bottom a dread of the avenging parents inside oneself. The child will not then ask for what he wants or even take it when it is offered to him, because of his dread that if he does get what he wants, that is, as he feels, if he is greedy and all-demanding, his parents internalised in his mind will revenge themselves upon him. So again it is safer to be hateful and to throw things away, or to say that they are bad and not wanted by him, not worth having.

Clearly related to this is the dread of the envy of other real people, such as brothers and sisters. Knowing one's own envy, as we all do in our hearts even if we deny it, we dread that of others. The only safe thing is thus to have nothing that can be envied, no sweets or precious things, not even health or success. It is better always to be the one who is overlooked or disliked or despised by the rest of the family; this is less dangerous than their secret envy would be if one was gratified. And one brings this

about by defiance or meanness or bad temper. For example,
the very small child in a large family quite often feels like this,
although it is only in some cases that it becomes an acute problem.
At a time when he is leaving his baby foods behind and begins to
look for the food which the older brothers and sisters and father
and mother are eating, what they eat, as well as their speech
together and all they can do, may have magical value just because
they are theirs; yet in his mind he dreads his wishes to take them,
steal them, or even to receive them if offered to him, since he
attributes to the older members of the family the same uncontrollable greed which he feels in himself, and fears them
accordingly. So it is better to turn away and want nothing, or to
refuse to be fed, to receive nothing from them. This attitude
is often carried over from the food which his elders eat to their
possessions, status, and skills. Occasionally this becomes a
settled persecutory anxiety; it is very strong in adults of the type
who become ill after occasions of success.

At all ages defiance and rebellion may be used as a means of
testing reality, as well as bringing upon oneself the punishment
that one secretly feels one deserves and needs. Hate is then
developed as a defence against the fear of parents and other
external persons and powers, the internal avenging parents being projected on to external authorities in home or school. This
is a normal way of response at various periods of childhood—
especially from eight to eleven years. It becomes abnormal only
when it is excessively developed and continued. Much of the
small child's defiance too, springs from this need to test his
parents, to see whether they are what he fears them to be in
his phantasy, and what they will do to him if he actually
becomes destructive and hateful.

Another motive for defiant, stubborn or destructive behaviour
at different ages is the need to confess, to bring to the notice of
the external parents the secret bad wishes which the child feels
within himself. He cannot trust his parents, his real parents,
unless he feels that they know something at least of the secret
bad things inside him. This is one of the motives in the small boy
for using swear words, or at a later age for compulsive stealing
or destruction of a kind that is bound to be found out. Under the
stress of this need, the child can only feel at ease if he is sure that
his parents do know of the danger they are in from his secret (and
mostly unconscious) greed or destructiveness. In acute cases,

whether with children or adults, friendliness on either side is felt
to be merely a deception and therefore very dangerous. Love and
tenderness are then wholly banished.

Again, hate and defiance are used as a defence against helplessness, the helplessness which may lead to frustration. This is
intimately bound up with the child's tendency to identify himself
with the "bad" parents rather than with the good ones, because
it is the bad parents who are felt to be really powerful. This is an
omnipotent attitude, arising from despair.

In a boy patient of mine, of seven to nine years, during one
phase of his analysis, this mechanism of identification with the
"bad" parents, and an omnipotence arising from the utmost
despair always showed itself in his voice. In manner and voice,
whatever he was doing at the time, he became simply "Punch",
as we know him in the traditional Punch and Judy show. It was
quite extraordinary to hear the "Punch" voice suddenly appear
and reveal the pleasure which Punch is represented as feeling in
his cruelty to Judy and the baby, the glee and the gloating in
power and destructiveness. I came to realise in the analytic
work, however, that when the boy spoke with this "Punch" voice,
he was not merely showing me his pleasure in destructiveness,
such as the real pleasure he had felt when he had actually teased
and hurt his little sister at home, but also the utmost despair, the
intense pain he felt at not being able to make his sister better or
to help his parents in their financial troubles and personal
quarrels. His despair was so great that the only thing he felt he
could then do was to identify himself with the powerful, cruel
father and so at least enjoy himself. [1]

Most of the defences we have been discussing operate in
everyone at different levels of the unconscious mind. This will
perhaps have been clear to you in what I have already said.
E.g. the fear of the adolescent regarding his sexual rivalry with
his father may lead him to turn away from home in defiance and
contempt; the little girl's rivalry with her mother for the possession of a baby may cause her to be rebellious and difficult.
Deepest of all in every person, however, are the anxieties arising
from the primary relation with the mother, from desire on the
oral level. In analytic work we find that obstinacy, contempt,

---

[1] Note (1947). This is the same boy as is described in the paper on "Property and
Possessiveness", where his anxieties and defences against fear are described in a
different context. See p. 41.

defiance and hatred are ultimately bound up with the anxieties relating to these earliest desires: the greedy love of the mother's breast as an ultimate source of pleasure and goodness, the wish to eat it up and incorporate it, the dread of the strength of such desire and the attributing of the same intense and uncontrollable wishes to the breast itself and to the mother. This fear that his greediness will destroy his mother leads to an intense dread of desire as such, which at times in all children, and habitually in some, is dealt with by tantrums, refusals, rejections and obstinacies, often openly connected with the feeding situation. In analysis we find that these early feeding difficulties link up with other types of defiance, obstinacy and hatred. Development is continuous throughout, and a full understanding of the later types of extreme defiance, such as delinquency, cannot be attained without taking these earlier situations into account. We have noted how the incidence of temper tantrums is highest in the second year and in most children tends to lessen and disappear as these earliest anxieties become worked over and modified and the child finds other ways of dealing with them.

To sum up briefly: Psycho-analytic studies show that rebellion, defiance and hatred may arise in children either from fears of bad feelings: envy, aggressiveness, revenge in oneself or others whether actual persons or the internal phantasied parents; or from fears of good feelings—desire and love, the need to give and help, guilt and the sense of obligation. In most cases there is a fluctuating combination of these defences in various situations and different levels of the mind. Most children and young people during development have recourse to these defences from time to time and to various degrees. The final flavour of a personality depends upon the way in which this or that particular mode of dealing with the internal problem tends to be weighted or fixed by external circumstances—perhaps by repeated experiences of an unfavourable kind. The differences between people as we know them in daily life are entirely a matter of degree and emphasis, not of an essential nature.

Let me illustrate some of my points now by a few examples considered in somewhat more detail. A little girl of six years of age, for instance, usually a child friendly to everyone, playing happily with younger children and co-operating with the grown-ups in her kindergarten school, suddenly seems to change her character, showing extreme defiance and hatred of the adults, tormenting the younger children and being unhappy and difficult generally. It turned out on enquiry that her mother had gone away for a period to nurse a relative's child. The little girl was staying with her father at the grand-parents' home and owing to unavoidable circumstances actually sharing a bed with him. When after six or seven weeks her mother returned, bringing with her a gift of a doll baby, the child showed instant relief, the necessity to be defiant and full of hatred disappeared, and she became again co-operative and friendly.

On the basis of analytic experiences, we should be justified in saying that she could not stand the absence of her mother and her jealousy of the other child to whom her mother was devoting herself, along with the great stimulus of her unconscious desire for her father stirred up by the circumstances of their sleeping arrangements. This whole situation filled her with guilt and anxiety, which could only express itself in behaving as if all the grown-ups were cruel and tyrannical and must be defied and hated, and all other children were rivals to be tormented.

Here is another example of a girl in whom the hardness and defiance were sustained much longer, and indeed seemed to become settled characteristics. From the middle years of child-hood—eight or nine years of age—up to the time of her marriage in her middle twenties, she appeared an utterly selfish and hard person. She gave no help to her mother in any way, seemed entirely self-seeking, had apparently no love for children or those younger than herself, and hardly any women friends. From analytic experience, again, one would surmise that this hardness and rebellion against all the canons of decent behaviour in her home arose from her great anxieties, repressed and denied, about her mother's health. From the time when the daughter was seven or eight years of age, the mother had a very severe, incapacitating and continued illness. She did not in external fact make demands on the daughter, indeed, in the opinion of friends and relatives, she over-indulged her; but watching mother and daughter together, I had no doubt that the child was terrified of the demands implicit in the mother's illness and of her own sense of guilt and responsibility. She really felt that she *ought* to devote herself entirely to her incapacitated mother, by giving up her profession, her leisure and indeed her life, to make her mother better. It may have been that in spite of the indulgent attitude of the mother, there was more of an unconscious demand on her part than she realised, but certainly whatever demand was there, real or phantasied, the daughter could not allow it to have any influence over her, and literally never did anything for her mother, but defied her and showed an utter lack of consideration.

In this particular case, the girl's character finally took a much more favourable turn than had seemed likely. Her mother died in the daughter's early twenties, and the daughter was later married happily, and has become quite an attractive and pleasant mother with a degree of maternal feeling which has surprised herself as well as others. It would be very illuminating to know the inner history of this change, but this could only be disclosed by analysis, for which no occasion arose. As a rule women who have such a bad relationship with their mothers either do not marry or are unhappy if they do, and are not at ease with women friends either.

Another minor example is from a young woman patient in analysis: it happened that going down a lonely street, she passed an old woman who was alone and had been taken severely ill and urgently needed succour. She was obviously poor as well as ill. My patient, like the Levite and the rich man, deliberately passed by on the other side of the street. The terror and anxiety which she felt when she saw the old woman's need led to her taking no notice and walking as far and as quickly away as possible—it was too overwhelming. She felt she was alone in the world but for an ailing old woman, who would take from her all that she herself had of health and goodness and comfort. This hard callous behaviour arose from her hidden anxieties, as in the cases mentioned of children who show defiance and lack of sympathy because of their unconscious fears.

Here is an example from childhood again, a girl who throughout her school years was characterised by obstinacy, noisiness, insubordination, seeking after boys, occasional stealing. At seven years she ate chalk (just as some younger children insist on drinking their bath water). She used in school to blow her nose very loudly in order to annoy a woman teacher whom she much admired and loved. In early adolescence she became an intellectual rebel against everything her father believed in and had frequent feelings of utter despair, with strongly marked suicidal tendencies. In her analysis it became clear that the motives for these characteristics were very complex and included most of those which we have already referred to. The outstanding influences were, first, that her mother had died when she was about six years of age, after a long and severe illness in which the home had become disorderly and unhappy. The child felt herself responsible for all these distressing happenings, especially as they followed upon her jealousy at the birth of a younger sister when she was about three years of age. Below this were many earlier anxieties connected with her love of her mother, her fear of her desire for her mother's exclusive love and attention and thus of the envy and hatred of her older brothers and sisters; and her still earlier anxiety that her own love and desire had damaged the mother's breast by its greedy quality.

In one short lecture I cannot hope to have made all these points or examples clear and convincing to you. It is only possible to hint at the complexities which may be behind this type of troublesome behaviour in children. One point, I hope, you will have realised; we are not justified in blaming the parents wholly for all the defiance and rebellion or other difficulties of their children. Sometimes the parents are at fault and circumstances or methods of dealing with the children need to be changed. But the complexities of human nature itself set bounds to our hopes and aims and may make our children difficult even when we have the best will in the world towards them. Not all our human wisdom and good will can avoid the conflict which arises inherently in the child's early and imaginative life. To understand this conflict a little further is surely a help to tolerating their difficulties; this understanding may not only ease the guilt of parents towards their children, but may enable them to deal more wisely with temporary troubles, and thus lessen the risk of rebellion and defiance turning into settled attitudes.

IV

PROPERTY AND POSSESSIVENESS[1]

(1935)

1. INTRODUCTION

I WAS invited to take part in this symposium on the assumption that some knowledge of the possessive attitudes of young children, and their behaviour with regard to property, would be likely to throw light upon the psychological problem in adult society. I believe this view to be a correct one, and that it is only on the basis of a *genetic* study of feelings and attitudes in the development of children's behaviour that we can come to understand the mental processes which become crystallized into adult sentiments, the institutions of property and the warfare of classes. That young children show a strong desire to possess material objects cannot be doubted; but a closer study of their actual behaviour, from infancy up to the time when the so-called "collecting instinct" appears in the middle years of childhood, will show that all behaviour relating to property is in fact a complex manifestation of many diverse psychological trends, including love, hate and rivalry with *people*. I do not believe that the relation between a person and a physical object, whether it be a toy, a utensil, a weapon, a dwelling-place, an ornament or a conventional unit of currency, is ever a simple affair between a person and a thing; it is always a triangular relation between at least *two* people and the thing in question. The object is a pawn in the game, an instrument for controlling and defining the relation between two or more persons. It may be a symbol of a significant bodily part of one or both of them.

This view of the complexity of the motives which enter into the overt attitudes of adults regarding material wealth is greatly strengthened by psycho-analytic experience. In the analysis of both adults and children, we find that their attitudes to material possessions frequently change a great deal during the course of the analysis. This change is often in the direction of a

[1] *British Journal of Medical Psychology*, Vol. XV, Pt. 1. A Contribution to a Symposium at the Medical Section of the British Psychological Society, 1934.

lessening of the strength of the wish to own, and a growth of the wish and the ability to love, to give and to create. Whatever the direction of the change, however, the fact that marked alterations occur under analysis, as the life history of feelings, phantasies and experiences is disentangled, makes it impossible to support the view that we are ever dealing with a simple "instinct of acquisitiveness" as such, let alone with "rational self-interest".

I propose to develop this broad conclusion by considering direct evidence, first, from the observed behaviour of young children in a group; and secondly, from the psycho-analysis of a boy in whom the craving for property and the wish for gifts was inordinately strong.

2. EVIDENCE FROM THE BEHAVIOUR OF YOUNG CHILDREN[1]

A group of young children (between two and six years) playing together in a free environment, which includes a variety of material for common use as well as a certain number of privately owned objects, will furnish countless examples of behaviour bearing witness to the strength and urgency of the naïve wish to own, the desire to have exclusive possession, or at least the biggest share or main use, of whatever properties happen to be the centre of interest. To a little child, the satisfaction of having things that are all one's own is deep, the chagrin if others have more than one's self very bitter.

The possessive impulse takes various forms. One is the direct wish to own an actual object, or to have exclusive use of it (which makes it "mine" for all intents and purposes). Any situation in which there is only one thing of a kind, an insufficient number of things for the group, or an assortment of things of varying sizes, will give rise to immediate tension as to who shall have "it" or "the biggest". With very young children it is often the mere size of the thing that counts, rather than its appropriateness; it is always the smallest children who insist on having the largest-sized tools, although they cannot manage them, and would get on much better with a medium-sized; the older and more experienced child will more commonly choose the more appropriate tool, and defend his right to that with equal tenacity.

A certain amount of teasing play will occur amongst children, in which they take away the property of others, not because they want to have that object itself, but because they want to

---

[1] This topic is also dealt with in *The Social Development of Young Children*, 1933.

rob the other child of it. This is a playful revenge, rather than a direct wish for actual possession. It has in it less of love of the object and more of hate of the other person.

Ownership is felt in things other than actual objects. Some children show a keen sense of property in the nursery rhymes and songs, or in gramophone records of a kind they have heard at home. No one else has the right to sing or hear these things without their permission. Again, children feel that anything is "theirs" if they have used it first, or have made it, even with material that belonged to the community. Sometimes they feel a thing is "theirs" if they have "thought" of it, or "mentioned it first"; and so on.

Some children will take it upon themselves now and then to act as dispensers of the public property and materials—the plasticine, the gramophone, etc. They may be quite well aware that the property in question is not "theirs", but they get a sense of power from deciding who shall use it and who not, or how much they shall have, trying to favour friends and exclude enemies. And if argument arises, the child who has constituted himself the master of ceremonies will often assert that the plasticine, etc., *does* belong to him, on the ground that *he* is "using it".

One of the commonest situations in which the possessive impulse is aroused occurs when a number of children want to use one of the larger pieces of school apparatus at the same time—the swing, the see-saw, a tricycle, the sand-pit. "Taking turns" is one of the hardest lessons for children under five years to learn. The young child cannot without much experience believe that "his turn" really will come in due time. All that he knows is that the others "have got it" and he hasn't. A few minutes is an eternity when one is eagerly waiting for a prized pleasure such as riding on a tricycle or a see-saw. Nor does one believe in the good-will of the others who are enjoying their turns first—one knows only too well how readily one would exclude *them* if one were allowed! Only the proved evenness of justice of a controlling adult will make a transition possible from the impetuous assertion of "I want it *now*" to that trust in the future which makes "taking turns" possible.

A particular incident occurring between two little girls of four illustrates the complicated processes that go to the development of a sense of justice in the use of property. One child was using the tricycle and the other wanted it. The latter complained to me that "A wants to have the tricycle all the morning, and won't give it to me". I suggested that B should ask A to let her have it after A had gone, say, four times more round the garden with it. B agreed, and I than added: "And perhaps when you've had it for four times round the garden, you would let A have it again for four times, and take turns in that way." B replied instantly: "Oh no! I shall have it more than four times—as many times as she has had it altogether—not just four—that wouldn't be *fair*, would it?" When the child argues thus she feels that if her enjoyment has to suffer limitations for someone else's pleasure, then she must have at the least as much as that other one. The logic runs: "If I cannot be supreme, we must all be equal. My wish for exclusive possession is tamed by my fear of the other's encroachments and the hope that if I admit him to equal rights he will take no more. But I cannot concede more." Equality is the least common multiple to these conflicting wishes and fears. If all are equal, no one has any advantage. And so "justice" is born.

Even in the simpler instances of the direct wish to own, it is plain that the relation to another *person* is a very important element. Neither the pleasure of ownership nor the chagrin of envy bears much relation to the intrinsic value of the things owned or coveted. Few objects, other than food when hungry, have an absolute and intrinsic value to little children, independent of what other children are having and wanting. What is so desperately desired may be wanted simply because someone else has it or desires it. A thing that has long been treated with indifference or contempt by the owner may suddenly assume great value in his eyes, if another person begins to take an interest in it; an ordinary object in the common environment, which has had no attention from the children, may suddenly become the centre of an intense struggle for ownership, if one of the children (especially the older ones), or an adult, shows that it now has value for him.

Turning to the situations which give rise to friendly co-operative play rather than to quarrels between children, one of the commonest and naïvest grounds for feeling friendly to other children (or adults) is gratitude for gifts received. In the frank and open-hearted attitudes of little children, both giving and gift are love itself. Much more is involved, however, than the simple desire for a material gift, than the wish to receive a gift as a sign of love. The child to whom a gift is offered shows by his response that he then feels *loveworthy*; and he who is denied, shows that he feels he has been denied *because* he is bad, because he is or has been hostile to the giver. It is this which brings poignancy to the child's gratitude for gifts, and bitterness to his sense of loss when he is left out of the giving. The gift is not only a sign that the giver loves and does not hate; it is also a sign that the *recipient* is believed to be loving, not hating and hateful. It thus brings him reassurance against his own sense of guilt and the pressure of his super-ego. The giver becomes *a good helper* (parent or ally) against the bad inside the child who receives. Whereas when he withholds, he abandons the child not only to his need, but to the rages and jealousies which that need and the sight of others' satisfactions arouse in him.

The obverse of all this is seen from the side of the child who makes gifts to those whom he loves. The wish to be *potent in giving* is very clear in much of the behaviour of little children. For if one has the wherewithal to give, one is indeed both safe and good. One is no longer the helpless ruling infant, dependent upon the gifts of others, and driven by helpless anxieties to rage and jealousy. One is now the omnipotent parent, full of good things, safe from unsatisfied desire, and all-powerful to help others (viz. one's children). It is more blessed to give than to receive, because to be able to give is *not to need*. It is (in unconscious meaning) to be omnipotently safe and good.

Even in the least complicated situation, where the value of the thing owned is intrinsic, the means of satisfying some (primary or derived) personal need, the actual wish to *own* it can best be understood in terms of power—or rather of *powerlessness*. "I want to own it because if I do not it may not be there when I need it, and my need will go unsatisfied. If another has it, he might keep it for ever. If I am at the mercy of another's will for the satisfaction of my need, I am helpless before it. Only if the means of satisfaction of my need is *mine*, mine to have and to hold, can I feel safe." Even here, there is a reference to other people, as potential frustrators, challengers or rivals. But, as we have seen, a great part of the value of those things which little children want to own is far from intrinsic. It arises directly from the fact that others have or want the object. And thus we enter the open field of *rivalry*. Not to have what others have, or to have less than they, is to feel small and weak and helpless. Not to be given what others have been given, or as much as they, is to feel shut out from the love and regard of the person giving. It is to be treated as not loveworthy. We can go further and say that the child who is not given what others receive (whether from playmate or adult) feels this exclusion to be not merely a denial of gifts and of love, but a judgement upon him. That is its chief bitterness, and the main source of the intensity of desire.

The ultimate situation from which the wish to own arises is that of the infant at the breast, whose satisfactions are indeed at the mercy of another's will. It is to the infant's sense of helplessness before the urgency of his need for love and nourishment, and the equally helpless rage stirred by the denial of immediate satisfaction, that we have to look for an understanding of the child's imperious wish to own.

To think of the motive of possession as a simple irreducible instinct is thus to miss its most significant aspect, viz. its intimate relation with the motives of power, of rivalry, of guilt and of love. It is essentially a *social* response, not a simple direct reaction to the physical objects which may serve individual purposes.

3. Evidence from the Analysis of a Seven-Year-Old Boy

Further light is thrown upon these overt group phenomena by the evidence gained from the psycho-analysis of a boy of seven and a half. This boy came to me for analysis because of an inability to learn, an inordinate craving for gifts and material objects, and a mildly asocial general attitude. His relations to people consisted almost entirely in asking: "Can I have that?" and "Will you give me this?" He was restless and inattentive, incurious and unable to learn at school, and generally unloving and unlovable. An incomplete analysis of two years changed this picture considerably. The excessive craving for gifts and objects was greatly lessened, he became more affectionate and more generally liked, able to learn more freely, to show more of the adventurousness normal to a boy of nine, and at the same time a greater capacity for penitence if his adventurousness gave rise to difficulties. During the course of the analysis, he constantly took away the toys from the drawer in the analytic room, and a certain amount of stealing occurred in his real life. A great deal of the play in the analysis was concerned with attack and robbery in one form or another. At one period we played out the Dick Turpin drama at great length and in detail. Sometimes I myself had to play the part of a thief, *e.g.* a black thief, an African, with black fingers, made black by black deeds of robbery. Briefly, the various *unconscious* meanings of material possessions and of his craving to get them, whether by asking or stealing, can be summarized as follows:

(1) The earliest bodily source of satisfaction, namely, his mother's breast. Unsatisfied oral cravings played a large part in his wish for objects. The boy had in fact suffered a good deal of oral deprivation in his early life.

(2) It was, however, not only the original primary satisfaction of both love and hunger, which he sought from the suckling; there was also a secondary need to find the "good" breast, as a re-assurance against his fear of the "bad" mother who had been spoilt by his own attacks of frustrated rage. These attacks had been made partly in phantasy, partly in real behaviour, by the means which every infant has at his disposal, biting, screaming, grasping, wetting and dirtying. The objects which he continually got or stole for himself, in later childhood, ceased each in turn to be satisfactory, as soon as he got it, because it then became the damaged breast which he had attacked. This was the deepest level of experience represented in the boy's craving for objects.

(3) His early disappointment at the breast, and fear of it as a result of his attacks, had led him after infancy to transfer his love wishes to his father and his father's penis. He then wished to attack and rob his mother of his father's penis, which she enjoyed in intercourse. This phantasy, and the wishes and anxieties associated with it, was played out in the analysis in, for example, the Dick Turpin play already referred to, but in many other forms as well.

The anxieties about the ruined mother led to a greater intensification of the need to get good from her, as a proof that she was not yet altogether destroyed and dead. The constant taking of the toys away from the analytic room mainly arose from the absolute necessity to have proof that I still had good to give him.

(4) Furthermore, these violent wishes to separate the parents, and to gain the father for himself, led thereafter to the urgent need to *restore* to his mother the things which had been taken

from her, whether the contents of her breast, milk and food, or of her body, the father's penis, her fæces and her children.

This wish to restore was very strong in the boy, and was played out in many ways in the analysis; *e.g.* by covering the walls of my room with drawings of telephones (some of them remarkably phallic in style). But since the boy's own penis had so often been the instrument of urinary attack upon his mother, it was felt to be incapable of itself giving good, of restoring, or creating. Hence the necessity to get good from some other source, to do good with. A "good" father had to be found to give the boy a "good" penis, as a means for restoring the mother. The boy felt he could not himself bear the guilt and responsibility, or endure the enormous burden of putting his mother right. If he tried to do this, he would himself be reduced to helpless penury and starvation, would be castrated, turned out and ruined. For a long period in his analysis he had much more faith in the possibility of finding a good father than a good mother. He made friends with men in the street, with bus conductors and lorry drivers, and openly wished to have a man analyst.

The anxiety to which the *good* impulses, the wish to restore and to create, led in this boy was enormous. It was strikingly shown in one particular analytic hour. There was a cupboard in the room where I kept my outdoor garments and my purse, and which was always locked. The boy knew that my purse and garments were in the cupboard, and had often begged to be allowed to open the cupboard and to have money given to him. One day he so managed circumstances with regard to his fare for travelling home from the analysis (a fairly considerable distance on the tube), that he was left with too little. He begged me to lend him a penny, to save a very long walk. I, of course, agreed, and opened the cupboard to get out my purse. The boy looked inside the cupboard; then at once said, "Good-bye—I'm going", and went straight out of the room and away without waiting for the penny. I did not at once understand what in the cupboard could have frightened him so much that he could not stay with me a moment longer, but had to leave immediately. I knew that he had had phantasies about marvellous things inside the cupboard, but it did not seem that the disappointment of these phantasies was enough to make the boy so terrified as to drive him instantly away. The next day he came twenty minutes late. After a good deal of play in which the theme was of my being an old woman with starving children, and having to beg or to play the piano in the street to earn my living, he spoke of a particular newspaper placard actually seen on the previous day, which ran: "Duke's son begs in street". He then suddenly asked me: "Haven't you *got* a coat?" This was the key to the overwhelming anxiety of the previous day. It was winter, but the day had been a mild one and I had come a very short distance to my consulting room and had not bothered to wear my coat. When I opened the cupboard the boy saw only a hat, and his instant belief was that I *had* no coat. And here was he borrowing (*i.e.* stealing, since he had no intention of returning the penny) from a poor woman who had no winter coat! Since he had been in analysis now with me for a year, had experienced the real benefits of understanding and felt he owed me a real debt, this notion stirred up an enormous terror that *he* would have to be responsible for providing me with a coat. As he was now in fact learning to play the piano, he would thus have to play it in the street, as he often saw a man doing in Wimpole Street, in order to pay for a coat for me. With many other threads which I cannot quote here, this led back to his despair as a small child, faced with the need to make good the damage he has done to his parents. His intense morbid craving to have things given to him was not only for the purpose of doing good with them, but even more to deny his guilt and responsibility, to prove to himself that he was still only a helpless baby who had never done anything wrong and who deserved only to receive.

In all these phantasies there were actual links with his real experience. The boy's father was a professional man with limited income and financial problems were of real urgency. From early childhood he had heard bickerings and mutual recriminations between the parents about financial difficulties. In his phantasy, it was his own early attacks upon his mother and his intense desire to obtain his father's love for himself which had led to these quarrels; and his own early greed and oral necessities which had made his parents poor.

Finally, the inhibition with regard to learning in this boy, whilst naturally very complex, had the following connection with his craving for material possessions. Learning is seeing and knowing, and to see and know about a thing is to want it; to want it is to damage it. So it is better not to learn. At the age of two years the boy had in fact been taken to sleep in his parents' bedroom, although occupying a room alone up to that time. He had undoubtedly been present at parental intercourse. He had not seen, but he had heard. He had wanted to see and to understand; and this wish had necessarily interfered with and separated his parents. Moreover, to see and know and learn is to accept responsibility, and since responsibility leads to the overwhelming task of restoring the poor quarrelling parents, it is better not to grow up, not to learn, not to know, but to deny responsibility altogether by being a child too little to learn, fit only to accept gifts from others. For him, the only alternative to this demand for material gifts was actual suicide, and the analysis uncovered definite suicidal tendencies, which were relieved by the later work of the analysis.

It will be remarked that in these notes I have said very little about the phenomenon of *anal fixation* in the love of property, whether in this boy or the children of the group described. That is not because I do not accept the fact of anal fixations operating in inordinate love of material possessions, but because I believe that, through the work of Melanie Klein, we understand a good deal more about the way in which these fixations arise.

It is possible to suggest that the desire for property, and in especial miserly cravings, owe their origin in large part to a shifting of desire *from* the living, human body to removable objects and lifeless material things, mainly because of anxiety about damaging the living bodies of persons. Sweets are craved instead of the breast because the person who gives them remains undamaged by the loss. Fæces, money and mechanical toys are feverishly sought instead of the penis, because these, if broken or ruined, can be thrown away and easily replaced. They can be taken without real bodily harm to the person from whom they come. The anal fixations represented in love of material possessions are thus strongly reinforced by displacement from the breast and the penis. The material objects embody and substitute relations with people. They are in the main a substitute for love, and counter the fear of loss of love.

In conclusion, I admit that I have not made any attempt to forge direct links between these deepest most personal and primitive feelings in the individual child, on the one hand, and adult social phenomena on the other. What I wanted to do was to challenge the crude psychological theory which uses a simple "instinct of acquisitiveness" as an explanatory notion for adult behaviour; and to plead for a closer co-operation between those most qualified to speak about the real psychological significance of material possessions to the individual, and the sociologists, who are concerned with the conscious sentiments of the adult, with large-scale behaviour and social institutions.

V

THE EDUCATIONAL VALUE OF THE NURSERY SCHOOL[1]

(1937)

1. INTRODUCTION

THE purpose of this pamphlet is to make clear the educational value of the nursery school for the young child. We shall focus our attention mainly upon the child's mental life and his needs as a human being, with wishes and purposes in relation to other people, and shall say very little about the service which the nursery school renders to his bodily health and growth. Much has already been written on the value of the nursery school in providing air and space and exercise, proper rest and good food, and thus remedying the serious lack from which so many children of the nursery age in our large towns suffer. Its function in these respects is now well established and widely acknowledged.

The wider educational work of the nursery school, however, is not yet so generally appreciated. This is true, largely, because our knowledge of the child's feelings and purposes, of his ways of learning and thinking, has itself only recently been won, and is by no means yet complete. We still have much to learn about the child's activities with different materials and his play with other children at different ages, and the various ways in which we can best foster his mental health. We now do understand something of all this, however, and are beginning to admit its immense importance.

We cannot, of course, sharply separate the care of the body from the welfare of the mind. Bodily health itself may depend as much upon the child's active play and happy relations with people as upon the right food and air and sunshine. Conversely, the child cannot be happy if he is starved and confined or suffers from lack of sleep. Whilst these two aspects of his development are thus intimately bound up with each other, it is yet possible

[1] First published in 1937 by The Nursery School Association of Great Britain: First Edition, 1937; Second Edition, 1938.

to focus our attention chiefly upon the one or upon the other, for the purpose of study. In this pamphlet we shall be concerned more with the child's personality than with his bodily hygiene; we shall refer to his body, not so much as an end in itself, but as an instrument of his feelings and intelligence.

The benefit which the little child gains from nursery school life is no longer a mere matter of opinion; it rests upon actual experience and demonstrable facts. General scientific knowledge of the child's needs of growth, and actual comparison of children who have attended nursery schools with those in the same general condition of life who have not, both provide evidence in favour of nursery school life.

A. *The scientific study of the behaviour of young children* has in recent years enabled us to understand the general lines of normal development from infancy to school life. Every mother and nurse and teacher has experience of her own to draw upon in trying to appreciate the needs of the children she deals with and coming to some opinion about children in general. But nowadays we are not confined to the narrow circle of our own experience. The knowledge and judgement of a great many observers has been pooled in scientific study. We have learnt *how* to watch and record the behaviour of children and how to arrange and classify the facts we have gathered, so as to come to more reliable and widely applicable conclusions about their development than can be hoped from the limited contact of any one of us, and especially from any one engaged all the time in the practical work of tending or teaching. We have learnt to observe large numbers of children both individually and in groups, either by giving them problems to solve under precise conditions, experiments and tests; or by watching their behaviour under ordinary conditions, in their daily lives, when they play together in the home and garden, and are at work in the school. We have learnt that above every other source of knowledge about children stands the study of their ordinary spontaneous play, whether in the home, the school playground, the street or the parks. The great educators taught us long ago that the child reveals himself in his play. In recent years we have come to understand more fully than ever before the deeper meanings of the little child's play. If we watch him when he is free to play as he will, the child shows us all that he is wishing and fearing, all that he is pondering over and aiming to do. He shows us what the grown-ups are to him, what attitudes he perceives in them, what his feelings are about them, and what are the happenings in the physical world which stir him to seek understanding and control. It is through his play that the child tells us most about his needs of growth.

Taking all these sources of knowledge together, we now have a considerable degree of understanding of the various aspects of the ordinary child's mental life as he grows from birth to the middle years of childhood, of its normal outline, its ups and downs, its movements in this and that direction, and the many and varied differences between one ordinary child and another. But we have still another important source of information. Many children do not develop straightforwardly with ease and happiness, but show difficulties of one sort or another in these early years. The infant welfare centres and the child guidance clinics all over the world have been now for many years helping these less happy children, those who are not able to learn as they should, do not talk at the normal age, cannot learn to read and write, suffer from tantrums, night terrors and fears, lie and steal, are destructive or aggressive to other children, or unable to play with them. These children, whose needs of growth have not been met by their normal environment and who need special help and remedial treatment of one sort or another, nevertheless teach us a great deal by their mistakes and unhappiness. In trying to help them we learn also what the lack has been, in what way the home or the school has failed them, and how we can avoid such breakdowns and difficulties in other children. By comparing these more unhappy children with ordinary children in home and school, we discover that the difference is not that ordinary children do not have any emotional troubles. The more we study the matter, the more we learn that emotional troubles of one sort or another are general and normal in the early years of childhood. The ordinary child in the good home, however, grows out of his difficulties. These other children suffer with a greater intensity and do not leave their troubles behind with normal growth. We are thus able to discover what are the ways of handling the difficulties of the little child which will help him to grow out of them, and what sort of attitude and behaviour in the grown-up increases and confirms the difficulties of development in the young child. Again, the study of the play of these more difficult children has provided another illumination of their needs of development. The unhappy child plays differently from the successfully developing child. He shows us the deeper sources of his trouble through his play.

Our study of these more difficult children who need special forms of help has therefore added to our understanding of normal development, and helped us to see more widely and deeply what are the child's needs of growth in the early years.

B. Besides this general knowledge, however, we are now able to draw upon the experience of many years of *nursery school practice* in different countries. For more than twenty years, a varying number of young children have been attending nursery schools in many parts of the world, and we have been able to watch and record the details of their development under these conditions. We can compare it with other children of the same sort who are not attending nursery schools. Careful comparisons have been made which show beyond question how much benefit in their mental life the nursery school can bring to little children. By comparing children from the same sort of family and the same general surroundings, of the same racial origin and the same degree of natural intelligence, we can measure more or less accurately the degree and direction of difference which the nursery school will make to their development. So far, all such studies have shown that children in the nursery school learn more easily, play more actively and thrive better in every way than similar children who have not this advantage even if they live in good homes. We can therefore look upon it as settled that the nursery school is a great help to the young child in his personal feelings and his intellectual life. It increases his happiness and helps him over the normal trials of early childhood.

2. A MASTER KEY TO THE CHILD'S DEVELOPMENT

In order to understand the service which the nursery school renders to the little child, we must consider what are his needs of growth during the earliest years after infancy. We have only to watch his play with a discerning eye, and to listen to his comments and questions, in order to realise how his mind is beset with *problems* of one sort or another—problems of skill, problems of seeing and understanding, problems of feeling and behaving. The appreciation of this central fact may be looked upon as the master key to the child's mental development. People have long sought such a master key, to unlock the meaning of the child's behaviour. Some have deemed they found it in the rôle of *habit*. Many teachers and text-books have emphasized the importance of habits and of training in the right habits in early education. And the child's readiness to learn particular sorts of habit, his general love of order and ritual, is indeed an important influence and a valuable aid in his life. But it is far from being the whole story of his relation to life. We cannot make the best use of habit unless we understand something of its true nature and function, of what it means to the child himself. Habit is one of the minor servants of life, the instrument of profound desires and purposes in the little child's mind. It is valuable *because* it helps him to solve some of his problems of feeling and behaving towards other people and towards his own body and his physical surroundings.

The ways in which life sets problems for the little child are endless. Let us look at some of the more characteristic problems which confront him—space will not allow us to do more than illustrate some of the main issues with which he has to deal during these years of early childhood.

A. *Problems of Perceiving and of Handling Objects*

These two aspects of the child's development—his sensory perception and his skill—used to be considered separately, and indeed as if they occurred in successive phases. Nowadays we know that they develop together and that the child is never concerned with his own seeing and hearing, tasting and touching as such, nor with his own skill, independently of the object upon which it is exercised. He is always, in his own mind, concerned with watching and trying to understand and to deal with things and people, the objects in the world outside him, which he so much needs to master and to comprehend. He is always trying to see things better, to make out the differences between table and chair, cup and spoon, apple and orange, the flowers and birds, the fire and the sun, the dog and the cat, the smiles and frowns of his mother, the faces of this person and that. His pursuit of these differences leads to the maturing of his sense discrimination and the storing of his mind with external knowledge, just as his pleasure in life and his wish to be like his parents and his older brothers and sisters leads to his zest in movement and the development of his skills.

Whilst the two-year-old child is well able to walk, and even to run, his balance and poise are by no means secure: he easily stumbles and is easily pushed over. His lack of balance and bodily security and his imperfect perception of sizes and distances naturally affect his feelings as well as his judgement. He is, for example, more readily afraid of other children, because he can so easily be pushed over, and his general sense of insecurity in life is the greater when he feels himself so unstable upon his feet, so unsure in reaching and handling objects. It is therefore not surprising that he shows immense pleasure in the attempt to master his own bodily mechanism, climbing up and on and over obstacles of all sorts, balancing and jumping, sliding, going up and down stairs. He loves moving in a way that employs the body as a whole. Later on, he is also fascinated by problems of manipulation, throwing pebbles, sand, pulling and pushing carts or horses on wheels, moving bricks about and arranging them in irregular masses, and occasionally piling them up and building.

Even at three years he seeks plenty of this general bodily activity, with now better balance and stronger movements. He delights in arranging objects with meticulous care, putting dolls neatly into their beds, tucking blankets smoothly in, arranging or piling blocks in definite patterns which have a clear meaning (for example, an attempt at an aeroplane or bridge).

One of the child's passions at two to three years is fitting sticks or blocks into holes of one sort or another. This impulse finds satisfaction in simple things like dropping pebbles into a pail, bricks into a box, tipping them out and putting them back again, as well as, later on, threading beads, putting blocks and sticks of different shapes into appropriate holes, and thus learning geometrical relations; moreover, just as the child loves putting little objects into larger, so he loves turning things out of containers —emptying drawers, pulling books out of bookshelves, tipping blocks or stones out of a cart.

Problems of pouring and dribbling, patting and digging and, later, modelling, with sand and water, give the child endless delight. In all the child's movements at two to three years, there is much pleasure in repetition.

A striking characteristic of the three-year-old when he is attempting to master some skill (for example, the use of the scissors) is the bringing of his whole body into play to aid the local movement: his tongue comes out or is twisted about, his legs move with his hands and arms, and his whole body may grow rigid in the attempt to master the particular movement desired. Only slowly, as the general bodily poise of the child increases and the manipulative movements of his hands and arms become more skilful, does he lose this rigidity of the body as a whole when attempting to perform some particular movement.

After three years, the child's power of manipulating such things as spades, brushes, pencils greatly increases. When running amongst other children, he can judge distances and speeds better, and is less liable to bump into them or to stumble and fall if others touch him when they are running. He still has enormous zest in the larger bodily activities, running, jumping and climbing, and needs plenty of opportunity for large free movement; but he has much greater capacity for the finer movements of hand and eye, involved in manipulating smaller objects. The bodily and manipulative play becomes less repetitive, the child's activities become more varied and he can play with several objects at the same time, combining them with definite meanings. He can respond to changes in the external situation more quickly and more fully, as, for example, when he needs to change his direction of running, or understand and obey an order or a suggestion, or seize a situation in the play of others. If anything is spilt or broken he will more quickly see what needs to be done to put it right. He can co-ordinate his muscles in the use of a tricycle or a scooter, and his use of all materials is more complex and more varied.

At two years of age the child still has very much to learn about spaces and distances and the relative size even of large objects. This was shown when a little boy of two, who loves to sit in a large packing case in the garden and pretend he is in a train, attempted, on one wet day when he could not go out, to fit himself into a small cardboard shoe box in order to enjoy his beloved game. He stood first on one foot and then on the other, doing his utmost to squat down inside this small box, as he did inside the large wooden one in the garden.

All the ordinary objects which surround the tiny child—chairs and tables, water and fire, sun and rain, cold and heat, animals and things, present problems to be understood. Every-day events which to us are a mere matter of fact—problems solved so long ago that we have ceased to remember they ever were such—are to him a puzzle and a challenge. A little boy of two, for instance, gazes out of the window on a cold winter day and sees the earth and houses and trees covered with a white sparkling powder. He says wonderingly: "Sugar", and is surprised to see "sugar" all over the garden and houses, until touching and tasting and the words of the grown-ups show him that this is a different sort of "sugar"—in fact, "snow". The same little boy is found powdering himself with a tin of Gospo. His wordless thought obviously runs: "Powder coming out of holes in the lid of a tin is what you put on the baby"—until he feels the grittiness of *this* powder, perhaps then sees that the colour is not quite the same, and is told that this is "Gospo".

Another two-year-old sees his older brother bring home a balloon from a party and pat it gaily upwards until it sails near the ceiling. The little one has never seen a balloon before, and gazes in astonishment, then runs to fetch his large rubber ball and tries to make this behave in the same way. *Why* will *his* ball not go up to the ceiling like his brother's "ball" does? The child seems to think the solution of this problem lies in the way his brother stands when he hits his "ball", for he tries to put his feet in the same position and assume the same posture as the older boy when the balloon sails up to the ceiling. This, of course, brings disappointment, and it is not until he can get hold of the balloon and *feel* the difference in its weight, and then perhaps notice the slight difference in appearance of the ball and the balloon, that he realizes that the solution lies in these character-istics, rather than in the way his brother stands.

A four-year-old boy playing with a bowl of water and little toy animals and men cries in distress when he sees his little toys "get smaller in the water", and sees his stick "broken" when he puts it in the water: "*Why* does it break my stick?" We adults may say that the toys do not really get smaller and the stick is not really broken—it only "seems so". We can "explain" the appearance; but to the boy, appearance is reality, and he cannot understand that his toys only *appear* to be altered.

The ordinary everyday world is full of such puzzling situations for the young child. All through the years from infancy onwards he is struggling with the discrepancies and bewildering incon-sistencies in the behaviour of things, with the puzzle of distances and sizes and shapes, of cause and effect. All these things have to be understood before he can hope to control them and satisfy his needs, and thus feel secure in a strange and puzzling world.

Even more full of problems to the little child is the behaviour of
the grown-ups. So many attitudes which to us are simple and
obviously right, so many values which seem clear and un-
questioned, are to the young child open questions, perhaps
bewildering puzzles, to be conned over and struggled with.
"*Why* won't people do nothing if people don't say nothing?"
asks a boy of three years—referring to the puzzling connection
between saying "Please" and "Thank you", and having good
things given to one. The child knows what the *feeling* of politeness
is, from the surge of love and consideration within himself, but
he does not understand the magic of this special formula, to
which some adults attach such a vast importance. Nor can he
readily deal with the many inconsistencies of adult behaviour,
and their to him incomprehensible reasons for giving or refusing,
for going or coming, for times and seasons.

In general, however, the young child is fascinated by what
grown-up people do. He loves to watch his mother cooking and
cleaning and washing, and wants to join in with her activities;
just as he loves to watch and to imitate his father, the bus conductor, the engine driver, the policeman, the postman. He is
struggling to feel and do as they feel and do, to understand their
aims and purposes and acquire their skills.

B. *Problems of Feeling and Behaving*

Let us now look at some of the problems of feeling and of
conduct which the child between two and six or seven years of
age has to face.

In these early years, the child's feelings are very intense. He has
little power of control and little understanding of the situations
which stir him. His affections are warm and passionate and his
delight in the presence of those whom he loves very great. Disappointment and the fear of loss arouse painful anxiety and anger.
At times he may be completely mastered by feeling, when he goes
rigid or lies on the floor and kicks and screams. Such times are
frequent in the third year, but tend to get less as he grows older,
partly through greater trust in other people and partly through
growing confidence in himself. Temper tantrums may be stirred
up not only by unexpected interferences by the environment, such
as not getting what he wants or being told to do something he does
not wish to do, but by disappointments at his own failures and
insufficiencies and exasperation at not being understood.

An important problem of personal life for children of the third year is the control of bladder and bowels. Whether or not there has been early training, children of this age are rarely quite secure in their control. Any emotional upset may express itself in a more or less temporary breakdown in cleanliness. The child's feelings about his excretions and his failure in controlling them, may be very intense. He may show acute anxiety, ex- pressed in screaming, great obstinacy, or in phobias of the pot or the lavatory. Difficulties in feeding and idiosyncrasies about food are common too, and are again an index of acute emotion. Both feeding difficulties and troubles about cleanliness are an expression of the child's feelings about people, and can never be understood as merely local or physiological matters. Nor can they be dealt with in simple terms of habit. To overcome them the child needs not only specific training, but, even more, the general help of a happy, sound life and the opportunity of varied play with other children.

The child of this age has very little power of co-operating with others. The three-year-old loves to be with other children, but only gradually does he come to feel them as equal partners in his own activity. The very young child naturally turns to his mother or to a nurse or other adult for attention, protection and love, seeking a warm personal relation. He finds it difficult to share the services of his beloved grown-up with other children of his own age, his chief attitude to them being one of rivalry and hostility. He will more readily be friendly to older children but is suspicious and hostile to younger ones. He may have attacks of acute shyness either with grown-ups or other children. To- wards the middle of the fourth year he begins to develop a strong wish for independence and is more ready to play happily and actively with other children. Under three he will rarely play for long with more than one other child, and three remains the commonest number of children playing together up to five years of age. In their love of a grown-up, children of this age are very possessive, just as they are of toys. The wish to share with others develops clearly only after this period. Throughout this period, however, there is an increase in the amount of play with others and more varied ways of joining together. The frequency and size of social groups increases. Children play together for longer periods and a larger number will join in in one activity. It is rarely that more than four children sustain a common activity, but very often five or six others will come in and move out of the group according to their changing impulses, perhaps joining with one group now and another a few minutes later, or going off to play solitarily and then coming back to watch or join in again with the first group, and so on. The four-year-old child's attitude is, "I want someone to play with me". The attitude of the child of five or six is, "I want to go and play with the others".

Group play becomes by degrees more active and more varied, the different rôles fitting into each other and showing more individuality. After three and a half, children are less dependent on adults, they turn to them for protection or approval and love less frequently, since they are becoming more confident in their active play with other children. They show less suspicion and less aggression towards others. They become capable of more tenderness towards younger children and of a protective and helpful attitude.

The very young child is often greatly afraid of his own hostile impulses to others. When he feels an intense surge of jealousy of another child, or anger at being interfered with by another child, he is also very troubled for the sake of the other child, and even very unhappy lest he should injure him in his anger. If he lacks the experience of playing with others, he is unable to measure the extent of his own control. If his positive attitudes to others are not strengthened by real experience, his distrust of himself and fear of his own hostilities remain unmodified. Later on, when the ordinary school years come, the child who has not had the experience of play with others is in a very different situation from those who have learnt, on the one hand, that it is possible to shout and run and sometimes be angry and jealous, without doing too much harm and, on the other, that other children are friends and helpers as well as rivals. The very small child is liable to demand an impossible standard of goodness and perfection from himself and to feel bitterly disappointed and anxious if he fails, if, for example, he should be clumsy or angry. Active social life with others gives him not only confidence, but a sense of proportion.

In his struggle with his own desire and urge, his own love and aggression, his own weakness and insufficiencies, the little child has recourse to many different ways of ensuring love and protection from others and lessening the tension of his feeling. One characteristic of these years is the occurrence of phobias—specific

5

fears of many sorts, such as biting insects and animals, dark shadows and moving wind, the coalman, the soldier or policeman, being bathed or having one's hair washed. Such fears in the little child are manifold. They are very real and intense to the little child, and often quite unmanageable. What he gains by them, however, are the love and protection of the grown-ups and the feeling that it is the animals which bite, the coalman who is dirty, not himself.

To help him grow out of his phobias, as out of his tantrums, the child needs experience which will foster his trust in his own power of being clean and loving, sensible and controlled like his parents, help in learning how to make things instead of spoiling them, how to protect instead of attacking, how to trust his own love instead of being *compulsorily* defiant and obstinate. Play with other children in surroundings that develop his affection and his skill is a great help in this direction.

Play with other children gives the child confidence in himself, no less than in his little friends, and not only helps him to feel less suspicious and aggressive to other children, and therefore less dependent upon the grown-ups, but by giving him the delights of active sharing and helping him to discover the way in which he can carry out his own practical or imaginative pursuits with others lays the foundation for a co-operative social life in the later school years. The child finds there are many things he can make with the help of others and many varied rôles that he can play with them that he could not carry out alone. All his creative and artistic interests are sustained and furthered by companionship with other children. The experiences of a child in a small group under happy conditions are infinitely richer in every direction than those of the solitary child or member of the very small family in the private nursery or garden, and those real experiences of sharing reciprocal satisfactions increase the child's belief in himself and his acceptance of life in general.

C. *Problems of Language and of Understanding.*

At two years of age the child is immensely interested in words and the use of words. He longs to be able to express his wishes and his ideas in words, to communicate his impressions of things, to ask for what he wants, and in general to have the intimate contact with other people through speech which he sees the grown-ups or older children have with each other. If we watch his face when he is listening to conversation and note the intensity with which he will try to imitate the talk of his elders or his exasperation when, through lack of words or faulty pronunciation, he cannot make us understand what he wants, we can see how strong is his desire to master this marvellous instrument of living. The ordinary child of two years of age is beginning to use words in combination; his sentences consist typically of a noun and a verb, although he will still use single words that have the function of a sentence. But most intelligent children are rapidly acquiring a vocabulary, and they develop a passion for naming, asking, "What's this?" "What's that?" all day long. Not only so, but they make immense efforts to put all their experience into words. For example, the mother of one little boy recorded how he would spend almost the whole of his day in making a running commentary on everything that happened and all that he remembered of his own or other people's activities. Many children, when they are left tucked up in bed at night, can be heard going over the experiences of the day, either in a string of single words or in attempts at a sentence, sometimes appropriately used, sometimes imperfectly understood. One can hear their pleasure in speech and the zest with which they try to make it intelligible. Many children of this age, however, are still afraid and silent and need the stimulus of play and companionship and of talk with the grown-ups to enable them to master language.

Where their store of real words is inadequate, children may invent their own, or will speak in expressive rhythms a hotchpotch of words and phrases, fragments of adult conversation. Children of this age usually understand a great many more words than they use, as is shown by their response to stories or commands. Intelligent children from cultured homes will naturally have a much larger vocabulary than duller children or those from homes where books and papers play very little part. Moreover, children who are not talked to or played with by the grown-ups or older children are poorer in speech at any given age than those who enjoy the stimulus of conversation.

Children's inventiveness is often shown in language. For example, two little girls of two-and-a-half and three-and-a-half had an amusing game of saying "Beetons on you" to any grown-up friend whom they liked. As they said "Beetons on you", they attempted to pick off some small imaginary object (beetles? or buttons?) from the garments of the approved grown-ups. These two children loved abbreviating words: strawberries became "strawbs"; "dogs' mercury" became "dogs' merc". Many children of two and three invent onomatopoetic expressions, e.g., when one child says, "It's raining?" another listens, and remarks: "Pit-patting".

The love of repetition in movement is paralleled by the delight in jingles, in nursery rhymes, in chanting and in spontaneous rhythmic expressions of everyday experience: "And I came home, and Daddy came home, and Johnnie came home", and so on.

Apart from differences of circumstance and of natural ability, the child's feelings play a great part in his speech development. Some children become inhibited in their learning and use of words, or develop special speech defects such as stammer, because this function is charged with intense emotion. Any unhappiness or conflict or temporary difficulty in the home, such as fear or jealousy of another child, the loss of a nurse or a beloved grand-parent, too frequent change of surroundings, or physical illness, may bring some check to normal speech development. A happy life and good relations with parents and brothers and sisters play a great part in fostering the child's use of language, whether for learning or art. Many words which to us are neutral may become highly charged with emotion to the little child, perhaps through some misunderstanding; as when a little boy sees some Scotch soldiers wearing kilts and hears the word "kilt" as "killed", and not surprisingly develops a terror of all soldiers he passes.

As the child grows from three to five years, his vocabulary is greatly extended and his capacity for expressing his wishes, his commands, his experiences and his opinions grows very rapidly. His sentences become longer and more varied in their construction. His talk is still, however, mostly an accompaniment to his building or drawing or painting or digging, his play with dolls and his make-believe. Meal-times are favourable to an interchange of talk, too. It is only in the most intimate contact with activity and actual experience that he begins to talk freely and to exchange ideas. He has little power for sustaining conversation as such, and needs the opportunity to talk with people who talk well. Grown-ups, or older children who will listen to what he has to say and respond appropriately are of far more value to him than specific lessons in clear speech. It is under the stimulus of wishes and emotions that language develops most freely and fully. At the beginning of this period children often talk about what they are doing without expecting much reply, but genuine discussion and even argument about what is going on do occur—always, however, in some practical play situation.

Intimately bound up with the development of speech is the growth of the child's power of reasoning. It is only as he learns to use words that he can effectively draw upon the experience of other people and deal with problems less immediate and concrete than those involved in actual handling of material. The puzzle which faced the little boy who saw snow for the first time was clarified for him by giving the word "snow" to mark the distinction between this white powder and the white powder called "sugar". Reasoning in words begins with intelligent children in the third year. When, for example, the little two-year-old coming home from a walk on a wet day takes out his handkerchief to wipe the gatepost dry and his mother says, "I shouldn't do that—the wind will dry it", he stands thoughtfully for a moment and says, "Wind dry it, wind got hankie", he is recalling his previous experience and making a leap of constructive logical imagination to solve the problem of *how* the wind can dry the gatepost. The same little boy sees a signal go down on the railway line in which he is greatly interested. He jumps with delight and says, "Sigernal down!" And then presently, "Sigernal down —*man* put it down". And after a few moments' further reflection, "Man put it down—man got ladder, man put it down"—an excellent piece of reasoning, drawing upon previous experience by means of verbal logic.

Throughout these years verbal logic, whilst always very simple, very concrete and immediate, yet shows continuous development. The child is constantly attempting to master the problems that concern him by drawing upon other people's experience in the generalized form of words. From three years onwards he seeks verbal explanation more and more eagerly. His earliest questions are, "What's that?" Then presently, "What for?" and a little later, "Why?" In the "why" questions of the four-year-old and five-year-old, we see the most intense effort at ordering experience in a logical and reasonable way. "Why doesn't the ink run down out of my fountain pen when I hold it upside down?" "How can the hippopotamus get down into his tank when his little back legs are so far from his little front ones?" are typical attempts to resolve the puzzles which confront him.

The power to reason in words and to formulate his experience grows in the little child through the opportunity to talk, to ask questions and to make statements *whilst actually engaged in his practical pursuits*. A rich experience, freely discussed, is the only means of learning to talk well and to think logically.

3. THE CHILD'S NEEDS

Let us now consider in broad outline the ways in which the child's environment and the people in it can aid him in solving the many and varied problems of learning, of feeling and of understanding which life brings to him.

1. In the first place, we cannot begin to help the child in his major difficulties unless we are aware *how real his feelings are*, how human and how like ourselves he is, how warm his affections, how acute his anger and dread, how despairing his grief and his sense of insufficiency. No method of education based upon the notion that the little child is a simple bodily machine or a mere creature of habit and reflex response can sustain him in his deepest difficulties. Such notions have led many people in recent years to deny the child the natural expressions of love in tender caress and simple responses to his cries and wish for companionship. Above everything else, a child needs warm human relationships, and spontaneous feelings of friendliness.

Growth in skill and confidence and social understanding come through pleasurable satisfaction in movement, in the expression of his wishes and his friendly responses to others, in food that is pleasant to eat as well as nourishing and well-balanced. Joy and zest in life affect the child's posture, his digestion and his learning —just as much as do food and clothing and exercise.

2. Another essential for happy development is *real and active experience*. No one can solve the child's problems for him, only *his own* moving and exploring and experimenting, his own play with toys suitable for his phase of development, can advance his skill and learning. It is the answers to *his*, not to our questions, which increase his knowledge. His efforts to understand the activities of the grown-ups and, above all, his interest in the primary biological processes of the household—the shopping and cooking and preparation of meals, the washing and cleaning and use of fire and water—form the nucleus of his intellectual interests. From these develops his wish to read and write; his later understanding of number and geography and history, of literature and

the human arts, is rooted in these primary interests in the life
of his family and home.

He needs, thus, not only the opportunity to run and jump and
climb, to build and model and paint and count and measure, but
also the companionship of grown-ups who have the patience and
the skill to answer his questions when he cannot answer them
himself, and to provide material for his activities as they progress
and develop from day to day. He needs a *generous* environment,
generous in warmth of feeling, and in opportunity for activity.
He needs appropriate materials to work upon and an attitude
of encouragement and eagerness in those who work with him.

3. One of the basic needs of the young child is *security*. Without
security as a background of his life he cannot dare to explore
or experiment, to express his feelings, or to try out new relations
to people.

Security has many facets: (*a*) First of all, he needs order and
routine and rhythm in the plan of the day. Regular meals and rest
and tending are not only important for the child's bodily health,
they also have profound significance for his feelings. A rhythmic
pattern in the details of daily life, no less than in music and in verse,
mean life and love and safety to the young child. The child's
own habits of bodily hygiene have the same significance to him.
Habit eases the necessity for decision and control and is a relief
to the tension of feeling; but the possibility of building up good
habits in the child rests upon order and rhythm in the behaviour
of the people around him and in the general pattern of his life.
(*b*) Secondly, security means a *stable attitude* in the people who
are with him. If the grown-ups are changeable and uncertain,
he has to watch for their smiles or frowns with a painful intensity.
He cannot learn control of his own feelings if he does not know
where the wind will blow from them. He needs serenity and
constant love from mother and nurse alike. (*c*) Lastly, security
means trust in the power of the grown-ups to help him to control
his aggressive and destructive tendencies. He needs to feel that
they will not let him bite or kick or hurt them, nor spoil, dirty or
break up everything. He needs to know that they love him in
spite of his faults and angers, and that they will not revenge themselves upon him by severe punishments. Mere indulgence,
however, is no help. The child seeks control from the outside
just because he has yet so little control in himself, and becomes
so afraid of his own jealousy and anger and destructive wishes,

unless he is sustained against them by the grown-ups' decisions. If the grown-ups are variable in their moods, he feels that he can too readily act upon them and make them pleased or angry, and thus he becomes frightened of his own power. The little child loves to obey when obedience is reasonable and is demanded by grown-ups who also allow him freedom to play and who understand his constructive impulses. The right use of the prestige and power of the grown-up in maintaining justice and order and in fostering constructive impulses is as necessary to the child as is the chance to assert himself in appropriate ways.

4. *The opportunity for self-assertion and independence* is another of the needs of the child's development. He needs the chance to learn to feed himself, to experiment in play, to jump and climb, to renounce the protecting hand, to make his own mistakes. It is a great advantage if the grown-ups know something of the average age at which the developing skills appear, but equally important that they should realize the differences between one child and another, and not try to force every child to keep the same pace. It is also a great help to the child if the grown-ups in charge know something of the normal age for perfection of the various bodily skills, if they can see when a defiant movement is really an impulse of growth, a search for an independence which can be achieved because body and mind are ready for it, and when, on the other hand, it is an expression of inner unhappiness. The child, moreover, thrives better if the grown-ups take pleasure in his growing independence; if they do not merely say he "ought" to be feeding himself or putting on his own shoes, etc., but enjoy it when he can do so. Independence which is yielded to the child for love and for pleasure in his growth is much more valuable to him than independence which he wrests from his parents as a result of his tempers and defiances.

There are times when the little child needs comfort, bodily caresses, encouragement and solace. When his phobias are enthralling him, when his anxiety about his own destructive impulses is uppermost, or when he fears he may never see his mother again because she leaves him after he has been angry or dirty, *then* he needs unstinted love and comfort; when he is puzzled about things which he cannot understand by his own efforts, he needs our answers to his questions. But at other times, what he needs most of all is the chance to experiment and to discover, to seek the answers to his own questions, to turn his back upon us and solve his own problems. The grown-ups who are tending little children need to have a sense of fitness and proportion, to know when to give and when to withhold, when to see the baby in the child, and when to respond to the man that he is to be.

5. And thus we come to the major need of the young child— *the chance to play with other children*. As we have seen in speaking of his problems of feeling and behaving, it is only by the real social experience of togetherness and mutual play—by finding out that the dangers feared from contact with other children are not real, and the harm one can do to them is limited, whereas the gains in other directions are so real and positive—that the child can develop into a social being. Many of the little child's troubles in his feelings about the grown-ups are solved in his play with his fellows. It is, e.g., commonly found in the nursery schools that feeding difficulties disappear very readily when children have their meals in common, and the tendency to thumb-suck or masturbate is considerably lessened. Night terrors, again, very often disappear when children attend the nursery school. Appetites improve and physical health is greatly enhanced. Through the lessening of anxieties connected, for example, with the child's own sense of helplessness and smallness, his clumsiness, and dread of losing his parents if other children come, play with other children fosters the child's growth and sense of security and happiness, and overcomes the inherent difficulties of his development.

It is not the mere presence of other children, however, which will do this for him, but *active* social experience—the working through of the difficulties of rivalry and aggression through free play, the forming and dissolving of groups according to the interests of the moment, leadership and following, even quarrels and fights, provided these are not allowed to go beyond a certain point. The child can only attain independence of the grown-ups and confidence in himself and in his own gifts if he has the chance of active play with other children. He can only develop the arts of expression in language and art fully and freely if he shares these gifts with others. The two-year-old child still needs a close relation with a grown-up, and at this age, nursery school groups need to be small in proportion to the number of the staff; but even at two years, play with other children under favourable conditions is a great pleasure and support to the child.

If we were asked to mention one supreme psychological need of the young child, the answer would have to be "play"—the opportunity for free play in all its various forms. Play is the child's means of living, and of understanding life. Much has already been said about the child's delight in physical skills and the aid which these bring to his learning and understanding. Another aspect of his play is make-believe. He needs the opportunity for imaginative play, free and unhampered by adult limits or teachings, just as much as he needs the chance to run and jump and thread beads. It is in this regard that our understanding of the child's mind and the way in which he develops has deepened and broadened in recent years.

Even the two-year-old already shows evidence of a vivid imagination—sometimes in wordless games, sometimes giving us hints of what he has in his mind by fragments of talk. But he has so little skill in expressing his phantasies clearly and articulately that it is very easy to overlook them and to think that he is "just" climbing or running or sitting still when, in fact, he is climbing in order to be "as big as Daddy", running in order to "be" an engine or a dog, sitting still and sucking his thumb in order to imagine himself once again a baby in his mother's arms.

The two-year-old uses his own body for his imaginative play, since he has as yet so little skill in subordinating materials. But every now and then a child of this age will give us a vivid glimpse of the large imaginative world that lies behind his simple actions. A little girl as young as sixteen months, for example, has a favourite game of picking off some imaginary fragment—presumably of food—from an embossed leather screen in the dining-room, carrying "it" with meticulous care across the room between her finger and thumb and placing it alternately in her mother's mouth and her father's. A little boy of two, who has enjoyed having his finger nails cut, begs his mother to cut them again, and when she insists that she cannot do so since the nails are already short, he makes a movement as if turning some imaginary taps, draws on to his hands an imaginary pair of gloves and then turns to his mother, "Got more hands, cut finger nails now", thus solving the problem of his disappointment by this magical action.

The child under three-and-a-half will use cupboards, as well as stairs and cushions, in fact all the larger objects of his environment, as a means of imaginative expression. The most frequent form of play with dolls at this age is putting them to bed and tucking them up, taking them out, comforting them, and tucking them up once more with care and patience.

Already at this age companions or brothers or sisters are invented and talked to and played with, and it appears that such imaginary companions are intensely real and vivid to the child himself. They share in a tea-party, for example, just as do the dolls or the teddy bears. Some little children become completely absorbed in the phantasy of being an animal: perhaps for three months on end they will "be" the cat or the dog, and insist on being treated in the proper way; or they will be Mr. So-and-So, "the man with spectacles on," "grandfather", or the tram conductor, and although their play will show very little appropriate detail, we can see from the child's voice and expression and gestures that he himself is lost in his feeling of identity with the person he is acting. Indeed, he seems to be more fully absorbed in this identity with the imagined person than an older child, who can work out the details in a more articulated way.

How little distinction the child of this age can make between what is real and what is pretended is shown when a boy of two years and nine months asks the older friend who is playing with him to "be cross and scold me", and when she responds very mildly he takes it so seriously to heart that he weeps and hides from her. It is only towards the end of this period that enough distinction develops between reality and pretence to make it possible to tell him ordinary fairy stories—those stories which are such a great pleasure to the older child but too real and too intense for the younger one.

The imaginative play of children of three to five years is extremely vivid and rich in expression. Every object in the environment will be pressed into service for make-believe play, which will be largely occupied with the reproduction of the typical situations of life—father, mother, children, washing, dressing, cooking, cleaning the babies, going journeys, defending the family against dangers of wild animals, giants and ogres; and with the externalization of the child's own feelings about himself and other people. Wild animals will represent the child's anger and greed and fear of punishment, just as the loving mother and babies and kind protective father will represent his belief in love and the goodness of parents. A great variety of experience is now represented. The dolls' house in which several children can join is much enjoyed, and co-operative play with different children filling out different rôles begins to be entertained. By six years of age the child is representing most of the every-day grown-up activities which he sees around him. There is a great passion for dressing up and long-sustained dramatic activity. The child becomes intensely absorbed in this dramatic make-believe, but nevertheless one can see the distinction between what is imagined and what is real growing clearer and more secure in his mind. However vividly he throws himself into his part it is clear that he now realises that it is make-believe.

We have come to see that the child's spontaneous make-believe play has two fundamental values to him. In the first place, it is a great stimulus to his intellectual growth. When he pretends to be father or mother, bus conductor, ploughman, engine driver, his play creates actual situations which lead him to remember and observe and compare and reflect upon his real experience, and which cause him to turn back to the real experience and look at it again and understand it further, so as to be able to make his dramatic play more vivid and more true to life. When, for example, half-a-dozen children are playing at father, mother and babies going for a train journey, and have arranged a row of chairs and are acting out the journey itself in the train, and the youngest child, impatient to be at the journey's end, jumps out of the train and says, "Here we are!" the oldest of the group, who is acting the part of the father, says in a stern voice, "Don't be so silly—we haven't got there yet", we see how his wish for dramatic similitude will stimulate the reflections of the younger ones on the realities of making a journey by train.

Again, make-believe play develops in the child the sense of past and future. He recalls his former experiences and envisages what *may* happen in order to solve the immediate problem. In general, he exercises in his make-believe play the characteristic human function of bringing the past and the future to bear upon the present.

Moreover, it is in his make-believe play that the child first glimpses the possibility of hypothesis, "as-ifness", without which no science is possible, no reasoning can be sustained. The very young child is quite literal-minded. If we ask a child of two years old, "What does Kitty say?" he will look round for the cat. It is only later that he can hold the image of a cat in his mind and remember what the cat does without confounding the image with the perception, only slowly that he comes to be able to work out the consequences of a hypothetical action without treating it as real. Yet to be able to hold a notion in his mind and develop its implications, "if so-and-so, then so-and-so", is an absolutely necessary step for his logical development. It is in his make-believe play that this capacity first shows itself.

The young child needs not only the chance to sit and dream his dreams alone, but to express them actively in his dramatic play with other children or with sympathetic grown-ups. It is by means of active dramatic play of this kind that he reaps the full value to his intellectual life of his imaginative processes.

We know, however, that make-believe play does far more for the child than this. It not only helps him to solve intellectual problems in understanding the behaviour of things and people, trying out now this, now that notion and developing it to its logical conclusions and testing it against the real facts, like the young scientist that he is, but also it helps him to achieve inner balance and harmony through the active expression of his inner world of feelings and impulses, and of the people that dwell in his inner world. When the child plays at being father and mummy and the family of babies, the giant and giant-killer, a wild animal and the hunter, the teacher and the pupils, the policeman and the bus driver, he is externalizing his inner drama—the various aspects of his inner personality—in just the way in which the creative artist in literature or painting does. The tiny child has not only his own conflicting impulses to contend with, he has also to deal with his first pictures of the grown-ups themselves as well as of the other children; his first notions of mother and father, the great, the terrible, the loving, the deserting parents. When he can, through the happy co-operation of other children, express these phantasies in active play, his inner tension is eased and a new equilibrium of mental health and happiness is attained. The solitary child, or the child with only one or two brothers and sisters at home, has less opportunity to work out his feelings in dramatic play. He is too close to the grown-ups then and has not varied enough contacts to give him ease and stimulus. In the nursery school, the greater number of children, the greater variety of personalities and the lessened pressure of external life enable him to come more freely to artistic expression and so to mental health.

Many of the child's interests in his actual environment and real life can only be satisfied in the larger group of the nursery school. When he wishes to construct and carry out activities of a shop, a hospital, post office, the train, he can do this better in the larger group. When his first interests in reading, writing and number work connected with these imaginative pursuits begin to appear, it is easier for the nursery school than for the mother in the solitary home to seize the golden moment and give him the technical help he needs.

5. THE SPECIAL VALUE OF THE NURSERY SCHOOL

In describing the development and the needs of the child from two to five years, much has already been said to point to the value of the nursery school. All that need be done now is to summarize these points and bring out one or two more clearly.

The nursery school is not in its essence a substitute for a good home. Sensible and loving parents in reasonable circumstances can and do meet the child's deepest needs. They give him love and security, understanding and sympathy, pleasant intercourse and happy play. There are many homes which fail to meet some or all of these needs, and where the home is ill-equipped or poor or the parents stupid or unhappy or, in some way, lost to the child, the nursery school has to make up for these lacks. That it can do so astonishingly well is shown by the way in which children from the slums, from the depressed areas or from broken homes, thrive when they are taken into the nursery school. But its prime function is not to take the place of the home: it is to supplement the normal services which the home renders to its children and to make a link between the natural and indispensable fostering of the child in the home and social life in the world at large. The nursery school is an excellent bridge between the home and the larger world. It meets certain needs which the home either cannot satisfy or cannot satisfy in full measure, and it prepares the child for his later life in school in a way which nothing else can do. Even children from a large family, so rare in these days, find support in the nursery school. In the larger family, the two-year-old or three-year-old often feels displaced and neglected when a new baby arrives. The nursery school, where he can make his own little friends and have his own life, is a great help to him in such a crisis. Conversely, the only child or the child from the family of two or three, gains the companionship he so much needs.

Speaking from the educational point of view alone, two-year-old children undoubtedly thrive in their homes, provided their homes are what they should be. The two-year-old still needs an intimate relation with one grown-up and does not easily tolerate the rivalry of a large number of other children. Towards the end of his third year, however, even where his home is ideal, he begins to need a certain amount of companionship with other children, and a well-staffed nursery school, where he can play with a few children of his own age or a little older, is a great help to his development. Those who come from poor homes in narrow streets, those who suffer from lack of nourishment or badly chosen food, those who long to play with other children and are alone in a family, will prosper greatly in a well-run nursery school even at two years of age. Whatever the home conditions, it is desirable to let a child from two to three years and onwards have some period each day in play with other children; and this is most easily provided in the well-equipped and properly staffed nursery school.

Let us now sum up briefly the many advantages which the nursery school offers as compared even with the ideal home. Any one of these benefits may be found in superior homes, but very rarely if ever are they all found together, except where two or three families living under very favourable circumstances join forces to provide the special conditions which very little children need, thus creating a nursery school.

1. *Space.* Space to run and throw balls, space to allow for the larger play apparatus—ladders, balancing boards, the climbing frame, boxes to jump from; space to trundle carts, to try out the scooter and the tricycle, space to shout without worrying the grown-ups and the neighbours, indoor space for wet days, as well as the outdoor playground and garden. Little children need space, both for their physical efforts and so that they shall not be too much in each other's way and annoy each other by contact or noise. To be boxed up in the small nursery or sitting-room of the ordinary middle-class villa or superior cottage is a very trying experience for vigorous, healthy children of three to five years of age and a source of great irritation and nervous strain. Space has in itself a calming and beneficent effect.

2 *Appropriate play material.* There is much play material needed for developing balance and poise and skill, for the first essays

in artistic expression and constructive handwork, the first attempts to understand number and space relations, and all this is far more easily provided for the group than for the small family. Moreover, much of it is better used in common than individually. The child's intellectual growth and social poise very often depend upon his having the right material at each successive phase of development, the right means of expression or of understanding at the moment when he is ready to create or to learn. The provision of the right material involves much knowledge of the growth of children during these years, knowledge which very few parents possess. Most parents rely upon the commercial toy-shop for their choice and thus waste not only their own money but the child's purposes. Nor can they as a rule easily provide the wide variety of constructive materials and the toys embodying an appropriate intellectual stimulus. This can, however, easily be done in the larger group, and it is part of the technical equipment of the nursery school teacher to understand the play material needed for each phase of growth.

3. Children need not only the right play material, but skilled help in their own efforts to learn and understand, and in their struggles with their anti-social impulses. To know what is the right word to say to the shy or inhibited child, the angry and destructive child, to have the right answer ready to an intellectual problem, to see when to introduce the child to a new piece of number apparatus, to understand when to interfere and when to leave alone, when to check defiance or stop a quarrel, and when to allow the child to solve his own problem, when to encourage and when to remain silent, is not a wisdom that comes simply by nature. Certainly it rests upon natural qualities. The nursery school teacher no less than the mother must have love and sympathy, natural insight and the patience to learn; but children need more than this in their struggles with the many problems we have glimpsed. They need true scientific understanding as well as mother-wit and mother-love. The nursery school teacher can often help where the mother would fail. On the other hand, the good nursery school teacher will see the problem from the mother's point of view as well and can often help her as much as the child. She is not there to take the place of the mother, but to serve both mother and child. Very often the intensity of the child's more difficult feelings about his mother and his brothers and sisters is lessened by the mere fact of having a friendly

nursery school helper as well, especially if she is a person of knowledge and insight.

4. *Companionship.* Enough has already been said to show the various ways in which the child's play with his fellows, with children older and younger than himself, in pursuit of his imaginative or his constructive activities, eases his psychological problems and fosters the development of his personality. The wider contacts both with adults and with other children ease the pressure of feeling in the child's relation to his own parents and to his brothers and sisters, and make for balance and harmony in the whole of his development.

In conclusion, let us say once again that the nursery school is an extension of the function of the home, not a substitute for it; but experience has shown that it brings to the child such a great variety of benefits that it can be looked upon as a normal institution in the social life of any civilized community.

VI

RECENT ADVANCES IN THE PSYCHOLOGY OF YOUNG CHILDREN[1]

(1938)

THE title of my lecture is too ambitious, and the necessities of time will impose a rigid selection on the topics with which I can deal. I shall only be able to speak of *some* recent advances. I shall take "recent" as referring to the last ten years, but in particular to the time which has elapsed since I had the privilege of addressing the British Psychological Society on this same subject early in 1932. The detailed work to which I shall refer has for the most part been carried out since that date.

I want first to discuss some general trends in child psychology of great interest and importance, and then to refer to certain specific studies. There will necessarily be many serious omissions, many most important studies both in this country and abroad which I shall not be able even to name.

The general trends I have in mind have carried much further certain tendencies which in 1932 I suggested were likely developments from the then state of things. To put it briefly, it could now be said that quantitative studies in child psychology are to a considerable extent approximating to clinical studies, both with regard to the methods and to the content of research. Quantitative methods are becoming more flexible than they were and less inclined to override or neglect complex facts for the sake of statistical and experimental simplicity.

One interesting recent contribution is a monograph published by the Society for Research in Child Development, on "Personality Development in Childhood", by Mary Cover Jones and Barbara Burks.[2] This surveys to 1936 all the facts of personality development in childhood which have been gained by objective methods, and discusses the present status of various methods.

[1] An Address given to the Education Section of the British Psychological Society at the Twenty-Sixth Annual Conference of Educational Associations, 1938. Reprinted from the Report of the Conference.
[2] Mary Cover Jones and Barbara S. Burks: *Personality Development in Childhood*, Society for Research in Child Development, Washington, D.C. 1936.

The existence of the Society for Research in Child Development itself indicates the trend of interests and of methods. Nowadays emphasis is on *development*, on a genetic approach to the problems of child psychology. There is a movement away from the measurement of traits as static units, whether by tests or by ratings, and a search for stable tendencies in a given, observable period of time, with definite patterns of variation, and as revealed in specific situations which are themselves to be studied, specified and regarded as a whole. Such research involves the study of the total organism, the child as a whole, and the study of the interplay of the various aspects of development within the developmental sequence.

Examples of the influence of this approach, and of the growing improvement in objective methods of research are very many. I can mention only one or two. The valuable work of Shirley illustrates these tendencies in many details. Shirley studied twenty-five children during the first two years of life, and the results of her work are published in three volumes.[1] She studied the child as a whole in the ordinary situations of his life as a whole, as well as in particular situations of observation and experiment. She observed and recorded every aspect which can be discerned within the total pattern of development, e.g., the locomotor sequence, manipulative skill, linguistic development, capacity for problem-solving, characteristic play at different ages, and the observable changes in personality, taking both age and individual differences.

One interesting example of her records is the way in which the child's attitude to other people in respect of timidity and shyness undergoes characteristic variations. There is a peak of timidity and shyness between the fifth and sixth months, and another at eighteen to twenty months. The first one is perhaps easy to understand, since it comes at a time when the child has learnt to discriminate between strangers and familiars. His visual perception, his perception of his mother or nurse as a whole, is now so advanced that he can distinguish quite clearly between her and a stranger, and he reacts towards strangers with reserve, withdrawal and shyness. After this period, he comes to be less afraid of the unfamiliar as such, and learns to distinguish between strangers and strangers, smiling at those, shall we say, who deserve it, and not at those who do not. The meaning of the peak at eighteen to

[1] M. M. Shirley: *The First Two Years*, 3 Vols. Univ. Minnesota Press, 1931, 1933.

twenty-four months is more complex, and I will not attempt to discuss it.

Shirley shows, too, how at every point the infant's social development is limited and then expanded by his development in motor ability, e.g., his being able (or not) to sit up, to look, to touch, to handle, to walk, to run; and so on and so forth.

Another example, this time in our own country, of work which illustrates the genetic approach is Lewis's study of infant speech.[1] In this interesting and valuable research, Lewis took phonetic records of all the utterances of a child from the earliest days up to the full mastery of speech, and noted the situation and the emotional setting in which each advance was made. He shows us, for example, how the first babbling impulses take origin in the sounds of comfort and discomfort connected with the feeding situation. The child repeats sounds which at first have been expressions of discomfort, turning them into a source of pleasure by repetitive patterns, thus creating the first rudimentary art-form. Again, he shows us how the infant passes through various phases in his response to the utterance of others. First he will babble back; then comes a period of passivity, when he appears to be listening rather than wanting to respond; then from about nine months onwards an imitative phase, when the utterance of others calls out a definite attempt to respond in like kind. In those and many other details there is an attempt to trace the patterns of growth, and to show the interrelation not merely between detailed aspects of speech development but between speech as a whole and the child's development as a whole, including his social relations with his father and mother, and his practical purposes.

Many fascinating results have been reached with regard to the interaction of the various aspects of development, in a number of researches. To take another instance from the details of this first year of life, it would appear that five months of age brings a definite crisis in development. Quite a number of interrelated changes then occur. Under five months of age, as Charlotte Bühler has shown,[2] there is a considerable predominance of negative attitudes and expressions of feelings in the infant, the negative feelings becoming gradually less and the positive ones increasing, until at about five months the picture changes, and

[1] M. M. Lewis: *Infant Speech*. Kegan Paul, 1936.
[2] C. Bühler: *The First Year of Lfe*. New York. Day, 1930

the positive outlook, with trustful attitudes and expressions of feeling, begins to predominate over negative attitudes (in the well-cared-for child). At about the same time, too, continuous directed activities and experimental play begin to loom larger than single reactions or random impulsive movements. This is obviously an important point in intellectual development. Another change at about the same time occurs in regard to the causes of crying. Under four or five months, children cry chiefly from physical reasons—pain, cold, too strong a light, too loud a sound, colic, uncomfortable posture, and so on. At five months and over, such things, naturally, may still produce crying, but social causes of crying begin to appear in addition. The child will now cry if, for example, his mother goes out of the room when he wants her to talk to him and play with him.

Still another change at about the same age occurs in the child's general attitude to the world. Under five months, the child cries chiefly because of external over-stimulation, things acting upon him which he does not like or cannot tolerate. He is a passive sufferer. After five months or so, he will also cry because he cannot do what he wants to do. For example, he wants to sit up and cannot manage it; he wants to reach for something and cannot get it. He cries because of the failure of his own intention, from the sense of frustration as an active, purposeful being. Five months of age thus appears to be a time of great importance, both in intellectual and social growth.

Another study which I shall content myself with merely naming, is Piaget's work on the moral judgement of the child. He has shown how that, too, passes through certain phases, which are interlinked with other aspects of development; the child's moral values change as his attitude to his fellows and to grown-ups changes and develops.

Taking all these advances in knowledge together, we are now beginning to obtain something like a reliable picture of the general phases of development in childhood, and the characteristic details of each phase. I have briefly outlined some of these in my little pamphlet on "The Psychological Aspects of Child Development",[1] and will not stay to elaborate them here.

It may be useful if I now refer to some of the actual comments on general trends made by experimental investigators themselves. In one passage Jones and Burks comment on the limitations of

[1] S. Isaacs: "The Psychological Aspects of Child Development." Evans Bros., 1936

former observational and experimental techniques, in yielding an integrated and consistent picture of the behaviour of the young child. They refer as one example to an investigation by Robinson,[1] an attempt to measure children's emotions by four techniques. Each one of these techniques was itself reliable, as shown by re-testing and by odd-even correlations, but the results from the four techniques showed a very low inter-test correlation. The techniques were (1) ratings of the children with regard to their emotional attitudes by nursery school teachers; (2) short sample observations of the children—fifty-one children—with regard to their facial and vocal expression in the playground; (3) ratings of the children on their emotional response in special experimental situations, designed to startle and to frustrate them; and (4) ratings of their responses on four of Marston's well-known tests for introversion-extroversion qualities. The correlations between the results of the four techniques were low, and Burks and Jones comment: "This may be attributed to a low community of function among the emotional responses, making necessary a great increase in the number of variables measured if we are to attain a valid index of emotionality. It is, however, possible that low inter-correlations arise merely through the incompetence of statistical procedure to reveal general factors which an analytical or clinical technique might expose. A child who is very reactive and emotionally expressive in the nursery school yard may become inhibited and 'poker-faced' when brought into a laboratory test situation. . . . A finer analysis might reveal that the child's playground behaviour was largely due to 'showing off', while his laboratory behaviour involved under-compensation for the same attitude. It is beginning to be clear that conclusions concerning the 'organization of traits' cannot be based solely upon mass correlations, if our interest is in the organization of behaviour in the individual."

Again, "it is significant that when people work *with* children, attempt to teach them, to cure them, to modify them or merely raise them, they nearly always hold some kind of working notion of total personality. A psychiatrist, clinical psychologist, teacher or parent who really conceived of the child as only a mosaic of specific habits would probably be very hard to find. Instead, the child is assumed to have a core of personality which 'explains'

---

[1] E. W. Robinson: *The Measurement of Children's Emotions by Various Techniques.* Univ. of California Library, 1933. Quoted by Jones & Burks, pp. 40–44.

and ties together many of his most diverse acts, which can to some degree be 'understood' by a sympathetic adult, and which changes its structure by gradations through the processes of growth and experience."

In this connection, Lewin[1] has attempted to avoid confusion between what he calls the "phenomenal" and the "genetic" aspects of behaviour. An embarrassed child, for example, may exhibit shyness or he may over-compensate and become loud-voiced and assertive. The phenomenal aspect would be the actual behaviour; the genetic or genotypic aspect would be the underlying feeling or attitude which is expressed in one or other of those ways.

Shirley, too, reported examples of this. She gives instances of one pattern of behaviour giving way to another while the underlying personality trend maintained its main direction. Three babies were described as "unco-operative" in the various tests and experiments. They habitually screamed during their tests until they learned to walk, after which they became the most strongly addicted of the children to escaping from the examination. First they screamed and later they ran away; but naturally the same attitude of being unco-operative to psychological examination underlies both behaviours.

Burks[2] herself made an interesting study of the predictability of children's behaviour in new social situations. She wanted to see how far people who knew children well would be able to predict what their behaviour would be. She got nursery school teachers to indicate what they believed the children's behaviour would be in three situations standardized by Marston. The first involved reaction to a stranger, the second, compliance in opening a difficult latch, and the third, self-assertion in the presence of desired toys. On reaction to a stranger, independent predictions of two teachers correlated to the extent of .82, which of course is much higher than is generally obtained between trait ratings. The correlations were very much lower in the other two cases, both as regards prediction and as regards the relation of the two tests. She suggests that the quality of a child's social feeling may be a pervasive and recognisable idiosyncrasy which can be translated into predictions of behaviour in new situations; but that

[1] K. Lewin: *Dynamic Psychology*. McGraw-Hill Pub. Co., 1935.
[2] B. S. Burks: "Personality Theories in Relation to Measurement," *J. Social Psychology*, 1936.

compliance and self-assertion, instead of being so described, must always be considered in relation to the individual child's interests and goals.

Jones and Burks sum up the whole question of theories of personality in this way: "The data adduced in favour of theories of specificity are not inconsonant with personalistic theories, but there are fragmentary data piling up by slow accretion and pointing towards a conception of integrated parts which fail to be accounted for by a specificity doctrine. Moreover, a personalistic theory, quoting Allport and Vernon,[1] has the advantage of defending the position of common sense."

Lewin, again,[2] commenting on the many researches which have been made to discover the effect of the child's position in the family, points out that "the statistical method is usually compelled to define its groups on the basis not of purely psychological characteristics, but of more or less extrinsic ones (such as number of siblings) so that particular cases having quite different or even opposed psychological structure are included in the same group." The "accidents" of the environment, which are ruled out for such studies, may really be the significant elements for the particular child; the decisive relation of the position of the individual child in the actual concrete total situation is abstracted. The fact of being the second, third or fourth child is nothing like as important in itself as the impact of the particular nature of the child above you and the child below you and the children all round you, the actual concrete psychological effect of the attitudes of those particular children, and of course the history of their common experience.

An important contribution has recently been made by an investigator who has become increasingly alive to the considerations I am putting before you. Lois Barclay Murphy has recently published a large monograph on "Social Behaviour and Child Personality".[3] In discussing problems of method she says: "For thirty years the canons of testing and the statistical criteria which tests have led to have been growing more and more elaborate and refined. Inevitably the attempt to arrive at statistical reliability led to a desire to find overt behaviour stable from one time to another, or repeated in identical form. Personality was thought of

---

[1] G. W. Allport and P. E. Vernon: *Studies in Expressive Movement.* MacMillan, 1933.
[2] K. Lewin: "Environmental Forces," *Handbook of Child Psychology.* Clark Univ. Press, 1933.
[3] L. B. Murphy: *Social Behaviour and Child Personality.* Columbia Univ. Press, 1937.

as a congeries of behaviour items, which varied in their dependability, but were significant for personality largely in terms of their
dependability. . . . Personality was about like a child's kindergarten Christmas tree, an outline with designs and decorations
of different shapes and sizes and colours pasted on. At the same
time, there has been a great deal of discussion about the 'whole
personality' in all the social sciences, yet the task of obtaining
research data which would permit of a scientific approach to the
whole personality, using statistical methods, has been so formidable as to frighten away most investigators. . . . Overt behaviour
may appear at different times and with different meanings for the
personality; therefore, psychological consistency (from the point
of view of the organism) does not necessarily produce statistical
or logical consistency from the point of view of the observer."

In her study she has made a valiant attempt to devise means of
observing all the complex facts, not merely of the children's
attitudes to her special topic, which is that of sympathy, the
response to a distress situation in another child, but the inter-
relation between this behaviour in the child at a given age and that
of the group of children among whom he is playing. She has
devised a series of experimental and observational methods which
are certainly much more adequate to the complexity of the facts
than anything else which has been done. She studies sympathetic
behaviour in cross-sections in the groups as a whole and then in
individuals, and she attempts to consider sympathetic behaviour
as an aspect of individual personalities seen as wholes, in addition
to the usual study of individual differences relating to age and sex.
Personalities are studied genetically also, to bring out developmental factors and processes of growth; and finally she observes
personalities as far as possible in their contexts, the context of the
immediate situation and that of the culture as a whole.

Murphy found, after a great many records had been taken
in various ways, that the degree of sympathy or co-operation or
fear or aggressiveness which the children showed was valid only
at the time the test was made and in the situation observed; there
is no way of arriving at a general trait of aggressiveness or fear
or sympathy or co-operation which will be valid for all situations.
For example, one little girl, Beulah, who during one year was
the youngest of the children in her group, had a low rank on all
the social responses but a high fear score. The following year,
when she was one of the older children of another group, all her

social responses were high, and with a greater trend towards aggressiveness than towards co-operation and sympathy. The picture had completely changed with a year's development and in a different group of children. Another little girl, Janet, whose picture in the first year was very similar, in the second year was at the top of her group for sympathetic response and co-operative behaviour, but low in aggressiveness. Another child, Patrick, showed marked aggressiveness in the first year, which hardly diminished in the second, yet there was a considerable increase in sympathy and co-operative responses in him during the second year. You have always to ask, therefore, in what situation and at what age and at what time the ranking was made.

Again, she asks what we know about any child when, taking all his rankings together, we have a general picture of his fearfulness, his aggression and his sympathy responses. We have to ask what the inter-relations of the different aspects are. There seem to be certain general influences; for example, a social child who is afraid for himself at a given period is also afraid for others. There are also specific relations; an aggressive child's sympathy responses are more apt to take the form of active interference, while in the case of a fearful child they are apt to take the form of warnings, protests or protection. Douglas, for example, who had a high ranking for aggression and a high ranking for sympathy, obtained his high rank for sympathy chiefly by defending children who had been attacked or hurt by others; Arthur was frequently anxious about the safety of others in situations which he himself feared, though they had no fear themselves; he was a timid child. A stable correlation of .40 was found between aggressiveness and sympathy in different groups, and it is suggested that a moderate degree of aggressiveness and sympathy indicate an outgoing responsiveness to the world as a whole; but that when aggression is very extreme, it may exclude both sympathy and co-operativeness—a conclusion with which anyone with analytical and clinical experience would probably agree.

Murphy is able to show what a wide range of behaviour occurs in individual children, and suggests that to understand the child you need to consider the *range* of behaviour rather than the traits in an abstract form. She gives many instances of changes due to changing circumstances and situations; for example, one boy who is excited and aggressive when another particular boy is there, is not so when that boy is absent. Again, when a child has done something to cause distress in others, then his attitude towards that distress will be different from what it is when he has not been the cause of the distress, and so on and so forth. There may be long-period changes in the child's behaviour, too. Murphy suggests that "a child's personality at any time may be defined in terms of the range of responses and the various nodal or peak points elicited by the range of situations to which he has been and is exposed."

I think you will agree that if these views and such researches are indicative of the general trend in child psychology, I am right in saying that there is an approximation of objective experimental and quantitative studies to the clinical point of view. Objective researches are now beginning to gather facts which are consonant with clinical experience, and which may help us to form a unified view of child development as a whole.

Some of the outstanding contributions to child psychology during the period we are discussing are various *"longitudinal" studies*, carried on with the same children over a considerable period of time. At this date quite a number of such studies have been made, some dealing with particular aspects of development and some with development as a whole. Observations have been carried on with the same group of children over a period of years, varying from two, by Shirley, to ten in the case of a recent study of intellectual growth by Freeman. In most of these longitudinal studies there are tests and re-tests as well as continuous observation. In America, several such researches have been carried out at the various Institutes of Child Welfare which have flourished in this period we are considering, and which, owing to their resources and endowments, are able to make use of several investigators on the one piece of research. When you have half a dozen first-rate investigators working together with the one group of children for five, seven or ten years, there is really a hope of arriving at significant facts of development, both in general and in particular.

One long-period investigation now being carried out at the Institute of Child Welfare at Berkeley, California, by Nancy Bayley[1] and others is concerned with general development of very young children. The same children have been tested and observed from birth to now six years of age, with regard to every aspect of their development, the tests used being combined from

[1] N. Bayley: *Mental Growth During the First Three Years.* Genet, Psychol. Mon., 1933.

Gesell, Bühler and others. This study has fully confirmed the view which I (among others) ventured to suggest even six years ago, namely that, in the first two years, the course of development is fluctuating and unstable, and prediction of future achievement from apparent ability in that period is not fully reliable. Bayley does not accept Gesell's view of the predictability of later development from the achievements of the child in the first two years. Her curves show considerable fluctuation in the first two years, these fluctuations becoming less marked, until at about two years development becomes much more stable, and prediction begins to be possible. Under two years the child is so sensitive to his experiences, and his emotional attitudes are so unstable, that his course of development cannot be fully relied upon to run smooth.

At the moment, another ambitious piece of team-work is going on at the Institute of Child Welfare at Berkeley, investigating the various aspects of development in adolescence. A group of boys and girls have now been studied for six years or so, from the age of eleven onwards, with regard to physical, mental, social and intellectual development, the appearance of the secondary sexual characters, the successive phases of behaviour in home and school, and many other points. A wealth of important new facts regarding adolescent growth, and the inter-relation of the various aspects in the history of individuals, is likely to result.

I want now to speak very briefly of fundamental advances made by means of the technique of psycho-analysis. Psycho-analytical research is, of course, essentially genetic in its approach, involving the study of a child's behaviour over a long period; and it is always concerned with the specific responses to this and that and the other situation, as well as to the general setting of his life; but, above all, it is concerned with the *meaning of the child's experiences to himself*.

In the last six or seven years, the chief advances in this field, mainly the work of Melanie Klein and Joan Riviere, have been in the direction of deepening our understanding of (1) the child's early love tendencies, early sympathy and identifications with his parents; (2) the complex interplay of love and hate tendencies in the earliest days, and the immensely varied modes of controlling, deflecting and diffusing the love and hate tendencies; and (3) the study of the "reparation" tendencies, the wishes and efforts of the child to make good any harm that his aggression and hate have done (in reality or in phantasy) towards those whom he loves.

In several important papers, Melanie Klein and Joan Riviere have developed these themes, and in a recent book, *Love, Hate and Reparation*,[1] they have shown in clear and simple language certain parts of our knowledge at this date on those topics.

It would be foolish to attempt any summary of this fundamental work, and I shall content myself with taking one or two concrete and illustrative points. These advances in the understanding of the earliest and deepest attitudes of the child, the interplay of love and hate and the reparation tendencies, have been achieved by taking seriously the very facts which the experimentalists often seem to regard as their special preserve, viz., the facts of the child's *behaviour* and of his response to his environment. The analyst does take the child's behaviour very seriously indeed, according full respect to all its details. He is concerned to discover what the *meaning* of any particular piece of behaviour in the child is to the child himself; not merely to record its existence and to see how often it happens, but to understand why the child behaved in that particular way at that particular time. And in the same way, to find what the meaning of this and that situation in the environment may be to the child himself.

Take, for example, the question of "tantrums". Objective studies have shown that tantrums occur more frequently at certain ages than at others, and that they are liable to occur more in certain situations than in others. The analyst is concerned to know what a particular tantrum occurring at a particular time and situation means to the child himself. That is, however, a very long and complex story, at which I can only hint. Let me cite some of the meanings which his fits of temper and excitement had for one little boy of four years with whom I myself worked. The boy was brought for analysis because he often had acute attacks of violent temper, with screaming and excited movement, on what seemed very slight provocation. Those tantrums had several important meanings to the child, but I will pick out only three. The boy's father was dead, and his mother had to work very hard trying to make up for the father to the child. She had a hard life, and did not always hide that from the boy. When the boy had these attacks of screaming and excited movement, he was first screaming for his father to come and help; he was using all the resources which the infant has—the loud voice and the violent movement—to call his father to the help of his mother.

---

[1] Melanie Klein and Joan Riviere: *Love, Hate and Reparation*. Hogarth Press, 1937

Secondly, he was acting out in his unconscious phantasy the feeling that the father *had* come alive again; the loud voice and the violent movements represented a powerful father, once more alive. But thirdly, in these screams and violence, he was also *fighting* the "bad" father, the father who did not help his mother, who ought to be there, but was dead. The father was "bad" because he was not helping the child's mother, because he *was* dead; and the child was fighting him, inside his own mind. In these and other ways the child attempted to deal with the terrific anxieties which the unhappy real situation aroused in his mind.

Here is another example of the way in which the details of the child's behaviour are regarded by the analyst with the utmost respect, and their full meaning sought. A boy of three and a half was brought to analysis, again for violent tantrums and abnormal dirtiness. At one year of age, he had lost his beloved nurse, on the birth of a baby brother. In the succeeding two years, he had no less than fourteen different nurses. He had been very dirty and screamed very violently in his anxiety and frustration, and to his mind, the successive losses of his nurse were the *result* of his being dirty and his screaming. To some extent, this was true. Several of the nurses had left for this reason, but it had not quite so much influence on events as he thought. For him, there was a simple and absolute casual connection between the two. When a parting with the analyst was approaching soon after he had begun analysis, because of the Christmas holidays, the child showed his dread of a further loss in this way: he took a little wooden doll, and got me to wrap it round and round very tightly with string, round both the middle of the doll and the neck and head and mouth. It was bound up tightly in this way with a long string, and then wrapped in paper so that he could take it home to his nannie. He was thus expressing his wish that I should give him some means of controlling his tendency to scream and to be dirty at home during the holidays, while he was not with me, in order that his present nurse, who has been with him for some time and is very good to him, should not leave him; and in order that I myself should come back to him. He already realized that through the analysis he would gain some control over these tendencies, and he wanted to be controlled, to be bound round, to be kept clean and kept from screaming during the holiday, lest his nannie should once again leave him, and that awful sense of loss come again. This small piece of behaviour thus had a very profound meaning for the child's whole past history, the whole of his attitude to life, and his future development.

I said that, in analytic work, we take not merely the child's behaviour but the details of his environmental situation with the utmost seriousness. We have to do that, because we find empirically that the work necessitates it. Here is a detail from the analysis of a man patient which will serve to illustrate this. He is a German, who came to England some years ago. He was psychologically ill, and came to me for help. In his analysis, it soon became clear that England stood to him for everything that was good and stable. It was not at first discernible why England and English things should signalise "the good" to him, since it certainly is not so with every German! One relatively superficial reason soon transpired, viz., his experience during the Great War, when the patient was a boy, and suffered very much from lack of food and the awful conditions in Germany. England was the unharmed, uninvaded country, where there still was good food and no revolution. The boy's natural conflict in adolescence was profoundly accentuated by War conditions, as well as typified by the War itself. And England stood as a symbol of all kinds of enduring good. This fairly soon became clear. Then, with more analysis, we came upon the fact that, much earlier in life, he had had an uncle who was a very learned and highly esteemed man, who had settled in England. This man stood in his mind for what was wise and good and creative and constructive, when he was a little boy. This fact not only helped to explain why England seemed so important to him, but showed also why the War had been such a bad experience to him; if in England he had someone who was so good and wise, then for Germany and England to fight meant to the child the most intense and acute family conflict. Only quite recently, with a good deal more work, did we come to what was even more significant, the deepest root in the child's experience of his feeling that England was good and safe and wise. When he was quite a tiny child of eighteen months or two years, his father had a German workman whose name happened to be "Englisch". This man was good in every way, and good to the child. If the boy, who was a lover of dolls, had a doll broken, he had only to run to this workman, Englisch, to have it mended. In particular, if the doll's eyes fell out, the child would immediately run to

Englisch to have the doll put right. This was the earliest and deepest root of the child's attitude of trust and belief in "Englisch" things. For full understanding, of course, we should have to ask why it seemed so fundamentally important to the child that Englisch could put a doll's eyes right; a story which would take us into the earliest history of the infant, and his own unconscious phantasies, his earliest wishes and anxieties and all his inner psychic life. And this we have no time to consider.

What I have been trying to do in this lecture is to indicate some of the trends in recent research into child psychology, and some of the extremely suggestive results of various studies affected by these influences, and to shew in general that there is a growing convergence of method and of conclusions between all investigators who are honestly concerned with real and living human beings, whose approach is genuinely psychological. We are beginning to see an approximation of clinical and of quantitative studies, which is bound to be immensely fruitful for the future.

VII

MODIFICATIONS OF THE EGO THROUGH THE WORK OF ANALYSIS[1]

(1939)

THE study of the various ways in which the ego is enriched and transformed during the process of analysis is a very large subject.

What I wish to do here is to open up certain aspects of the subject which in my view and that of several of my English colleagues are of fundamental importance, although they are only now beginning to be understood. In our experience the most far-reaching and most satisfactory modifications of the ego come about by means of the analysis of the earliest anxiety situations and the most primitive defence mechanisms. I need hardly say that this is not to be taken as meaning that the defence mechanisms belonging to the later phases can be neglected. The fact that I am not concerned with those in this paper does not mean that I do not think their understanding essential in the actual work, and in the total picture of psychic development.

1. CHANGES OCCURRING IN THE EGO

In a satisfactory analysis which is brought anywhere near to completion, the patient's ego alters and expands in many different directions. Some of these are as follows:—

(1) Sexual wishes, both heterosexual and homosexual, in their varying emphasis and individual colour and in their relation to the Œdipus complex, come to be accepted as an integral part of the mental life, and to find satisfaction either in a direct form or through various modes of sublimation.

(2) The capacity for bodily pleasures becomes freed and enhanced, as the masturbation phantasies are brought out and understood.

These phenomena are so familiar to us that I need not elaborate them here. That they can to-day be largely taken for granted

[1] A revised version of a paper read at a Symposium at the Joint Meeting of the British and French Psycho-Analytical Societies, Paris, April 30th 1939. Not previously published.

7

in any discussion among analysts does not mean that they have lost one jot or tittle of their fundamental significance, whether for theory or for practice.

(3) Bodily health improves as the release of feelings, the recall of repressed experiences and the reactivation and expression of phantasies in the transference situation gradually relieve the patient of the need to resort to conversion and hypochondriacal symptoms as a substitute for feelings, memories and phantasies.

(4) The sense of reality develops and becomes more trustworthy. This, too, has been a familiar theme in psycho-analytical literature, ever since Freud formulated his view of the reality and the pleasure-pain principles, and showed how they operate in the mental life. There is, however, a great deal yet to be said about the "sense of reality". It is not only a matter of judgement, but even more a matter of feeling. The ability to see things objectively is bound up with the distribution of feeling and feeling-tension.

The reality which the neurotic fails to appreciate is primarily a social reality, the real feelings and characters, the conscious and unconscious attitudes of other people. In the course of his analysis, the patient gradually becomes more able to see people as they are, in the complete setting of their lives, to tolerate their faults and deficiencies as well as to appreciate their gifts and virtues.

One very striking and almost universal change lies in the patient's judgement as to the relative goodness and badness of the two parents. We know how extremely common it is for a patient to see all virtues in one parent and all vices in the other. Sometimes indeed a patient thinks and feels almost as if he had had only one parent, the other being well-nigh obliterated, both in memory and in value. In such cases the relation to the actual parents has throughout been over-shadowed by the phantasy-figure of the combined parents,[1] a phantasy formed in the earliest phases of development and reinforced by many complex feelings and defences.

Analysis could be said, in a very real sense, to give the patient two parents, with regard both to his present-day life and to his memories; and it brings the power to feel and to act appropriately towards the two parents. The recovery of his feelings, not

[1] Melanie Klein discovered the infantile phantasy of the "combined parental figure" and discussed its importance for early mental life in her book *The Psycho-Analysis of Children*, especially in the chapters on "Early Stages of the Œdipus Complex" and "Anxiety-Situations in the Development of the Ego". (Hogarth Press, 1932.)

only in the present-day but also as experienced in his earliest past and then later on denied, distorted or forgotten, transforms the picture of his parents, brothers and sisters first presented to us, and yields a truer knowledge of them as they were in his earliest awareness of them. Moreover, the patient recovers and re-values his experiences with regard to other people too, other members of his family, friends, school-fellows, and acquaintances generally. These recovered memories of historic fact, and memories of his own earliest feelings and perceptions, enlarge and fill out his present-day ego, giving it depth, solidity and stability, and improving his present-day social relationships.

(5) The possibility of appreciating *external* reality better and reacting to it more appropriately is bound up with the growth of the ability to feel and understand *internal* reality, the world of feelings, phantasies and personal values. As Freud taught us, internal "psychic" reality stands between the individual and his appreciation of external reality. It is primarily the neurotic's denial of his own inner world which renders him unable to appreciate external reality. He becomes able to distinguish between inner and outer reality just in so far as he can bear to learn to know his own feelings and to appreciate his own phantasies.

I believe this to be just as true for the small child and even for the infant as it is for the older child and the grown-up. No one who sees the infant of six to twelve months watching the faces of those around him and responding instantly by smiles or frowns or signs of anxiety to the emotions portrayed on the faces of others can doubt that he has an intuitive awareness of expressions of emotion in other people, one which may become blurred later on, but is his natural gift in the early days. And if it becomes blurred, if he has to deny what he sees in the faces and behaviour of other people, whether it be anxiety, reproach, anger, coldness or greed, then this is because these external phenomena stir up unbearable feelings and phantasies which have to be shut off from the ego.

For the infant the mother's angry, sad or frightening face does not remain an external object; it has its immediate counterpart in his inner world owing to the power of the introjection mechanisms which are characteristic of the early mental life. The mother's angry face outside corresponds to an internal angry mother. The denial of the inner reality of the angry, sad or cold face in his own mind, and his own feelings towards such a face, lead to the denial of the external reality and to the impoverishment of the ego. In analysis, a recovery of these phantasies, feelings and memories leads to the expansion of the ego both towards the external world and towards the depth of the internal world.

(6) As these changes go on, there appears in the patient a general lessening of rigidity of feeling and attitude towards other people and towards himself, a lessening tendency to compulsive "repetition" of the early patterns of his life, a loosening of the obsessional stranglehold on emotion and wish; and there appears an increasing ease of adjustment and of capacity to respond to changing situations in external life.

(7) In general, there is a great enrichment of feeling, in depth and variety and spontaneity. Anxiety is very much lessened, but it can be more readily felt as such. Feelings of guilt, of fear, hatred and anger can be better acknowledged and better tolerated. And the capacity for feelings of love and tenderness, of sorrow and regret, is greatly enhanced.

The capacity to feel for and with others, to respond to their objective and subjective situation with true appraisement and sympathy, and to feel them to be people in their own right, gradually takes the place of the tendency to treat them as mere puppets in the patient's own life, mere sources of pleasure, reassurance, guilt or anxiety. Along with this goes a freeing of aggressive tendencies, which begin to find a more adaptive and appropriate mode of expression. Love and hate become not only freer, but better mingled and applied. And this gives a firmer texture as well as greater force and energy to the ego.

(8) In many patients the freeing of the inner world results in a capacity for creative pursuits of various kinds. The ego becomes able to tolerate phantasy life instead of suppressing it and to use id-impulses in a creative way.

I would emphasise here that the function of the well-developed ego is not only to control, but also to express. Its expressive is surely at least as important an element in its total synthetic function as its controlling aspect. The ego which is fully equal to the demands of life is in touch with its own sources, the world of feelings and of inner values. It can express and use its own impulses, is on good terms with unconscious phantasy, and can accept pleasure and enjoyment.

But to attain such an ego means a change in the inner world

itself, the growth of some belief in love and creativeness there, that is to say, growth of trust in his own impulses and in his introjected objects.

2. THE ANALYTIC BASIS OF THESE CHANGES

The width and depth and enduringness of these changes in the patient's ego depends mainly upon the extent to which we are able to analyse the most primitive defence mechanisms, those which are directed against the most primitive anxiety situations, the early oral phantasies regarding "bad" internal objects, the loss of "good" internal objects, and the relations of these phantasies and feelings to the earliest objects of love and hate.

The mechanism of manic control, as a defence against depression and persecutory anxieties connected with these primitive phantasies, is the main factor in bringing about rigidity of personality and paucity of feelings, as well as the denial and distortion of external fact, and largely contributes to faulty ego development in general.

In her many contributions to the theory of psycho-analysis during recent years, Melanie Klein has taken up the discoveries of Freud and Abraham with regard to the mechanism of introjection, and greatly expanded and elaborated our understanding of the complex psychic processes involved. It would not be practicable here to attempt even the briefest summary of the wealth of observations and unifying theoretical considerations which have now been brought forward with regard to this enormous psychological field. Reference must be made to the published papers and books of Melanie Klein and her collaborators.

What I wish now to emphasise is that these phantasies regarding internal objects themselves represent the most primitive activities of the ego. They arise during the earliest period of life, and are the first, the most pervasive and most enduring psychic elaborations of instinct and experience.

They are the product of the infant's mental activity at the time when his relation to objects (his mother's breast, face, voice, person) is dominated by his oral wishes, when his sucking, biting and swallowing impulses provide the pattern of his feelings and

---

[1] See for example her *Collected Papers* (1948) and *The Psycho-Analysis of Children* 1932).

wishes towards those whom he loves and needs, indeed, towards the world in general.

In my view, the observable facts of the infant's ego development during the first few months of life support the conclusion arrived at from the analysis of young children, viz.: that in the beginning, the oral pattern dominates the infant's perceptions and active responses to the external world, as well as the quality of his feelings. Other types of activity, other relations (looking, listening, grasping, etc.), derive their first impetus, their first cathexis from the infant's aim of sucking, biting and swallowing. Later on they become independent aims and independent satisfactions, but at first they are subsidiary to oral purposes. (Grasping, e.g., does not become an aim in itself before about nine months; until then, the infant, reaching out to grasp any object he sees, does so mainly *in order to suck and bite it*.)

In this phase of development, when the child's essential relation to the world—at first, entirely, then for many months, mainly—is that of a suckling, his sensory experiences of touch, kinæsthesis, hearing and sight, etc., his bodily pains and pleasures, his own feelings of satisfaction and dissatisfaction, of love and longing, of disappointment and loss, of hate and fury, are worked over psychically and unified, in the pattern of his own oral aims and impulses. He assimilates what he sees and hears and touches by means of his phantasy, his imagination; and his phantasy is in the first instance the psychic expression of his instincts. From the beginning phantasy embodies experience too—the earliest experiences of bodily sensation and external perceptions, held together and coloured by early instinctual aims.

At this time, too, when the child's perceptions of external reality are under the thrall of his oral aims, his feelings, his affective responses to his actual experiences of pain and pleasure, are at their highest level of intensity, of all-or-noneness. His desire, his needs are urgent, and frustration may be unbearable.

One sequence of processes initiated by frustration may be described as follows. Pain and fear of loss stir up uncontrollable rage and the wish to attack and destroy the breast which frustrates him, and which yet he longs for so intensely. But this wish to bite in hate and fury in its turn arouses further dread of loss, since it will destroy the source of pleasure. He feels helpless, both against the object which creates such love and longing and hatred, and against his own over-mastering feelings. And his love and longing and hatred and destructive fury may bring about an overwhelming dread of helplessness, of dependence upon loved objects, and a stifling of any feelings of love.

He seeks to lessen his dependence upon external objects, first by incorporating them, and then by retaining them. But if he has them inside himself, they cannot escape from his hate and fury any more than from his love and longing. He incorporates them, both in order to have them and love them, to draw their goodness from them and live by them; and also in order to imprison, punish, attack and destroy them. He wants to bite and swallow in both greedy urgent love and destructive hatred.

In phantasy, thus, the breast is inside him, inside his own body; the breast which he loves, the fount of all good, of life and love, the "good" breast; but also the breast which he hates, the breast which not only frustrates him, but which by his own destructive attacks upon it, has itself been made full of hate and evil and destructive impulses towards him. Thus first the breast, then the face and voice and person of the mother and later also of the father are felt to be active and moving inside him, whether dead or alive, loving or hating. They are *objects* inside him, objects of his love and hate, within his body. He loves and hates and fears them, loves to keep the good ones, but fears their destruction by the bad ones, longs to get rid of the bad ones, to "project" them back into the external world—as he expels his own fæces, with which he mainly identifies the bitten up, destroyed objects he has incorporated—but fears to let them out again, out of his control. At times he phantasies that with his excretions he has got rid of the bad destroyed and destructive objects; and for a time, now feels full of the good ones,[1] the good satisfying milk, the loving breast, the kind mother. But urgent bodily needs and desires arise again, and sucking, biting, swallowing the good breast, needing and demanding and incorporating the good mother, again destroys and loses the good objects; once more they are turned into fæces, once more they become bad and destructive inside him. In these phantasies he is subjected to attacks by the persons and parts of persons he has swallowed and taken in in greed or in hatred, and has made bad by his own attacks upon them.

---

[1] In this presentation of infantile phantasies reference is made mainly to the mother. The processes described, while primarily concerning phantasies about the mother, soon include those about the father and other members of the family.

One very important aspect of this situation is the feeling that it is his very need of good objects, his need of love and life, his greedy urgency, his dread of frustration and dependence, which itself destroys the good. Love and desire may thus come to be feared above all else, since love and desire are so intense, so consuming, and thus so destructive.

These are pre-verbal phantasies, and apart from analysis they find their way into consciousness and speech later on only in the indirect way of simile and metaphor, which largely frees them from their direct and personal meaning, and renders them innocuous to the conscious mind. Such phantasies sometimes find more overt expression in various products of art—which, often enough, cause offence and revulsion in the audience.

Now there are endless individual variants on this fundamental and universal situation. In the more or less normal person, the relative degree and specific forms of love and hate, the specific modes of maintaining a balance between taking in and giving out, between the inner and the outer worlds, between loving and hating, the specific phantasies regarding the nature of the internal objects and their relation to each other inside, may vary in great detail from individual to individual. In the work of analysis, one has to appreciate and bring out all the specific individual details of content and feeling, together with the relation of these details to the facts of early experience and personal history.

In those whose early greed becomes greatly overemphasised (whether by reason of constitution or circumstance), greedy love and hate become almost indistinguishable. In those whose case·is a little less than the worst, love may yet be feared more than hate, both because it is in itself so greedy and because it stirs up *uncontrollable* hatred—hatred reinforced by greedy love. Such persons tend to exploit open hatred (in its many forms of coldness, rejection, defiance, spite, cruelty, love of power, etc.), towards people in the external world—hatred which is measured and controlled and turned into a pleasure, as a defence against love which is uncontrolled, unmeasured, and brings endless pain and loss to the lover and the loved.

This exploitation of open hatred as a defence against the greater dangers of love and desire, towards actual people in the external environment, rests largely upon the projection of the terrifying internal objects into the outer world. In all patients whose ego has remained under the thrall of these primitive mechanisms, the distinction between the inner and outer worlds tends to be blurred. The external world has little existence in its own right; its function is mainly this one, of serving as a deposit of the most dreaded inner objects, and as a place where destructive impulses may be directed—in order to save the good objects, retained within. Such patients manage to retain their hold upon life, and some semblance of a relation with external reality, largely by turning their hate outwards, and thus preserving, but hidden away, denied, never drawn upon, a secret store of love and pleasure, a good unharmed breast and mother and father.

In her paper "A Contribution to the Psycho-Genesis of Manic-Depressive States",[1] Melanie Klein has to some extent developed her view, inspired first by Freud's work on "Mourning and Melancholia"[2] that phantasies about an inner world in which the loved objects are felt to be destroyed by the subject's aggression and by hated objects which threaten the self as well, underlie states of depression (depressive and persecutory anxiety). She went on, moreover, to show how in such situations the individual may have resource to the device of omnipotent control. If the objects can never be made good and whole again because unconsciously love is felt to be so greedy and destructive, the objects may have to be kept under rigid control.

This aim of controlling inner and outer objects is, according to Melanie Klein, part of the *manic defence*.

In her study of the negative therapeutic reaction, Joan Riviere[3] took up this concept of the manic defence and showed its special working in the persistent refusal of certain patients to get better. But in passing she referred to the widespread and comprehensive character of this defence, and the diverse phenomena to which it gives rise. She says: "The essential feature of the manic attitude is omnipotence and the *omnipotent denial of psychical reality*, which, of course, leads to a distorted and defective sense of external reality". After remarking that Helene Deutsch had pointed out "the inappropriate, impracticable and fantastic character of the manic relation to external reality", Joan Riviere continues: "The *denial* relates especially to the ego's object-relations and its *dependence on its objects*, as a result of which *contempt* and depreciation

[1] *I.J.P.A.*, Vol. XVI, Pt. 2 (1935).
[2] *Collected Papers*, Vol. IV, pp. 152–170.
[3] *I.J.P.A.*, Vol. XVII, Pt. 3 (1936).

of the value of its objects is a marked feature, together with attempts at inordinate *control and mastery of its objects.*" And again, after referring to the "immense importance" of the manic defence as a factor in mental life, she writes: "It is true that we have known of many of its manifestations and even had a name which would have represented it if we had known how to apply it— the word omnipotence. . . . We ought now to study this omnipotence and particularly its special development and application in the manic defence against depressive anxieties."[1]

It is this primitive and universal defence which, if unmodified, hampers and limits the subject's relations with people, with external reality and with his self.

The mechanism of manic control expresses itself in protean modes of neurotic character and faulty ego development, as well as of illness. It would be impossible to catalogue these phenomena, but examples which spring to the mind are: moral aggression, due to the projection of death and destruction upon other people, who must needs then be attacked; lack of sympathy and tolerance with others in distress or error, since those who are in any way injured or imperfect are felt to be too dangerous and must be controlled, kept at a distance and thus rendered harmless; artificially idealized love objects, in whom not the slightest imperfection can be admitted, since imperfection stirs up guilt and anxiety (this type of love has no warmth and can stand no strain); compulsive lying, since apparent honesty is itself felt to be a terrible lie, when the inner world is so hopelessly bad; conscious dishonesty having its roots in unconscious denial of the value and reality of anything: Don Juanism and over-sexuality which brings no happiness, with a constant greedy search for new objects of love and pleasure, since those already attained are soon felt to be valueless.

These and many other failures of true enjoyment, of feeling and of judgement in the ego ultimately spring from the need to deny and to control the internal situations of depression and persecution.

Only when the intense love and hate felt for the inner objects and the intolerable guilt and pain connected with their fate is experienced in the open, and the relation of these feelings to the earliest external objects and actual experiences is brought out in the transference situation, together with the particular expression

[1] Op. cit., p. 308.

of the manic defence in the individual patient, with specific details of the way in which he has kept these phantasies and feelings at bay, does the patient's ego expand, and the capacity for love and bodily pleasure, for satisfactory relations with other people and for creative work, fully emerge.

Apropos of some of the points which were raised in the preceding discussion I would like to challenge emphatically the view that *we* have to strengthen the patient's ego, to *make* it independent of the super-ego, to *make* the latter flexible, etc. *This is what happens*, if we understand what goes on in the patient's mind, i.e. his feelings and phantasies towards ourselves as analysts in the transference situation. The patient's ego does grow stronger and more independent, through his experiences in the transference situation. We do not need ourselves to have an active or an omnipotent attitude towards his ego.

In my view, what Freud taught us about the importance of avoiding a moral attitude to the patient remains as true as ever it was. Although as human beings we cannot help some feeling of satisfaction if, in the process of becoming well and capable of giving and taking pleasure, the patient also becomes a more useful and attractive person, yet as *analysts* we should not let ourselves act as his super-ego; nor should we behave actively towards his vices and virtues. We need *only* to understand and interpret them; and, I would add, to understand and interpret his virtues as well as his vices.

This last is a point of the very greatest importance. I know that there are analysts who believe that our task is to analyse only what is *un*satisfactory, "abnormal", "neurotic"; and that any feeling, character trait or behaviour which we consider to be satisfactory or "normal" should not be inquired into, not be analysed. I believe this to be fundamentally incorrect, both as a matter of theory and of practice. Theoretically, it seems to assume that there are no unconscious roots to what is "normal" or satisfactory, a view which cuts across the whole theory of sublimation, as well as Freud's discovery of the super-ego. There is surely *no* mental process, no aspect of the personality, which has not its genetic history and its roots in the unconscious. It would be utterly impossible to understand the meaning and etiology of a patient's symptoms or faulty character development by examining them alone, in isolation from the whole psychological history, the whole personality. Symptoms and character

traits, the useful and the undesirable traits, the normal and
abnormal aspects of personality, are always intimately intertwined in development and in unconscious significance.

From the point of view of practice, I believe it to be faulty
technique to attempt to confine our interpretations to what we
consider to be abnormal, and to judge that "*that* is normal, no
need for any interpretation".

The patient needs us to understand the whole of his history,
of his conscious and unconscious trends, of his personality. He
needs us to analyse him, not to judge him. Analysing him means
seeing the inter-connections between his symptoms and his ego
trends, appreciating what he himself accepts and what he rejects
of his own unconscious wishes, why his unconscious aims stir
up such anxiety that they have to be denied, displaced, repressed,
projected; or why they can be tolerated and built into his conscious
self. He needs us to understand the specific nature and function
of his anxieties at the various periods of his development, especially
at the various crises of his life. He needs us to see how his unconscious phantasies and anxieties are now being expressed or
dealt with; to see the specific connections between his earlier and
his later modes of equilibrium, his most primitive and his later
developed mechanisms, between his earlier and his later object
relations, in the Œdipus complex, and in his sublimations and
character developments.

Only in so far as we gain an understanding of the whole shall
we reach an adequate understanding of any part.

I have said that we need *only* to analyse the patient, and he
himself will then be able to bring about the new balance of ego
trends which results in the manifold changes we have been
describing. But I would emphasise again that we do need to
analyse the patient's whole personality, to bring out the unconscious love as well as the hate, the reparation tendencies as
well as the greed and destructive wishes. It is partly because so
much of unconscious love and reparation wishes find expression
in the so-called "normal" characteristics and in the sublimations
that it is essential that we should trace, as the patient shows
them to us, the unconscious roots of these traits as well as of the ·
failures and neurotic symptoms.

But we need also to see the complex hidden and distorted ways
in which unconscious love will express itself, the desperate ways
in which the psyche will struggle to maintain the life and safety

of its inner objects and of the self. The manic defence itself, for example, absorbs and contains a wealth of unconscious love and the wish to preserve the loved persons, though these are at the same time paralysed. We should never relieve the stringency of the manic defence if we saw in it only hate and search for power.

But whatever the picture of the unconscious may be, as it is revealed to us in the transference situation, our task is to accept it, to understand it and to put it into words for the patient, so that it can be worked over and modified by his conscious ego. If the patient shows that he is projecting upon the analyst at the moment the destructive mother or father in his inner world, or that he is terrified of his love for the analyst, because of its greedy nature and the disaster to which he believes it will inevitably lead, we help him more by bringing into the open these psychic facts and showing him how they came about, than we would do by hastening to assure him that it is only imagination, that it is unjustified, untrue, or that we are in fact kind and well-meaning. If we fulfil our true analytic task of giving adequate verbal expression to what he shows us, whether it be hate or love or fear, and whatever the concrete nature of the phantasy or memory— this in itself brings him the greatest help against his phantasies, the greatest support to his ego.

The analysis—through the transference situation—of these earliest anxieties and earliest defences brings about profound changes in the *unconscious* layers of the ego. There is not only an increase in the depth of the ego—the ego growing at the expense of the id and the super-ego, as we used to put it. There is also a qualitative change in the lower levels of the ego itself, with a re-distribution as well as a modification of primitive feeling. (This is, of course, always a relative matter; but the degree of it affects the extent and depth of the ego changes which we began by considering.)

This modification and re-distribution of unconscious forces comes about through the *experience* of love and hate and anxiety in the day-by-day work of the analysis. The projection in the transference situation on to the person of the analyst of the loved and hated and feared internal figures not only enables them to be brought to the touchstone of external reality, but is followed by the re-incorporation of these figures in a modified form, modified by the experience of the analyst's patience and tolerance of hate and aggression, together with his understanding of anxiety.

Love becomes diverted from its fixed and hidden unconscious forms and released to more adaptive and fluid conscious purposes. Love has increased at the expense of hatred and fear; security and trust, at the expense of doubt and disbelief. And thus there is more freedom of feeling and of action, more acceptance of internal and external truth, more belief in goodness and more capacity for enjoyment and constructive work. All this implies a great lessening of the need for manic defence.

One other point I would like to add. In stressing the importance of the analysis of early phantasies and the inner world, I do not in the least imply a *neglect* of external reality. I do not believe in the opposition in technique of emphasis upon internal and external factors. They are, in my experience, inextricably bound together. The child's actual experiences become interwoven with his inner world at every instant of his life. If it were possible to pay attention *only* to phantasy, we should not understand it. If we imagine we can understand the true meaning of what actually happens to the child, *without* taking into account what he brings to events of his own phantasies and feelings, we ourselves suffer under a delusion. Phantasy and experience may be momentarily separated in the direction of our attention, for the purpose of distinction and understanding. In actual life, both are always in operation. What we are always concerned with in our work is *the meaning to the child* of the person in question or the external events which impinge upon him.

3. ILLUSTRATIVE MATERIAL

The following brief references to a case history may serve to illustrate some of the conclusions presented in this paper.

Mrs. X. sought the help of analysis because she suffered from attacks of severe anxiety and various symptoms, including sexual frigidity. She was a married woman and had one young child.

When the analysis began Mrs. X. was in an acute state of anxiety. She had quarrelled violently with her parents about her husband. She felt that her parents were unjust and mean towards him. As it turned out in the course of the analysis, such quarrels were a recurrent feature in her life and whereas she made her parents responsible for them, it was in fact she herself who provoked them, usually by making use of her husband as a tool.

She seemed superficially fond of her husband and her child, but there was little deep affection or tenderness in her relations towards both. She had never experienced pleasure in suckling or tending her baby, in fact she had not wanted to have a child. She felt all along that there was a great deficiency in her attitude to her child and to her husband and she had a deep longing to be able to love her child and to be a good mother. As it was, her relation to the child was hedged round by rigid rules.

She showed a strong tendency to control and manipulate people and situations. She was full of hate against her parents. Neither had any virtues. She described her father as a tyrant actuated by nothing but sadistic impulses towards her. The fact that he was a distinguished author did not count with her, she took no pleasure or pride in his achievements, barely admitting them as a reality. She also had nothing good to say about her mother, e.g. she regarded her mother's attempts to make peace between father and daughter as a sign of weakness and deceit. She was always able to justify her hostility against her parents. The parents were well-to-do whereas my patient and her husband were poor. Mrs. X. demanded monetary help from her father as a matter of right. (This attitude, too, was part of her incessant need to dominate and control her parents.) She never felt that her parents gave her enough and in this way justified her greed and her feelings of revenge and hatred. At the same time she was extremely tied to her parents and emotionally dependent on them.

Some of the symptoms about which the patient complained at the beginning disappeared fairly soon in the analysis, e.g. her frigidity. But it took a longer time to effect changes in the realm of the ego. Progress in the ability to judge people and a more objective assessment of reality, above all in the capacity to understand people and feel sympathy with them, was slow. Whenever there was a step towards improved relationships, or an act of consideration or understanding of others, this was immediately followed by a violent reaction, of compulsive cruelty, hardness or obtuseness.

Gradually the severity of the patient's illness became clear. She not merely showed some hysterical and obsessional symptoms, but psychotic features also emerged.

In this connection I would mention that one of her recurrent compulsive actions was to pick out fæcal matter with her fingers at night, especially before having intercourse with her husband. The analysis of this habit which could be regarded as a perversion brought to light memories and phantasies, which showed the strength of her anal-sadistic impulses. In her phantasies fæces were weapons to attack her parents with, to ruin her mother's body, and the babies which she felt her mother to contain. This early hatred against her mother went back to grievances related to the feeding situation and had reached a peak during the second year of life, when her mother became pregnant. She was eighteen months old when her youngest brother was born. The sadistic phantasies related to this event and the severe anxiety stirred by it proved one of the most essential factors responsible for her sexual and emotional development. The new baby was felt to deprive her of her position as the youngest and most favoured child. He was the rival displacing her from her mother's love. To watch him feeding at her mother's breast stirred in her unusually strong oral grievances. She hated her mother for withholding from her the lap and breast which she herself desired and claimed as her right, and she hated her father for giving a baby to the mother but not to her and frustrating her in this respect also. The fact that the new baby was a boy roused envy of his genital, and his birth was thus felt as the frustration of all her wishes. It must be stressed that this reaction to the youngest brother's birth and the inability to overcome her jealousy and hatred can only be explained by the excessive strength of the child's sadistic impulses and of the guilt to which they gave rise. There are many children to whom the arrival of a new baby, especially at such an early age, is a traumatic experience, but normally feelings of love make it possible to accept the sibling as a companion and moreover to share to some extent maternal feelings with the mother. The excessive amount of fear and guilt in this little girl, however, prevented her from developing a constructive attitude and made her feel that the baby's birth was nothing but a punishment by her parents for her greed and hostility.

The persistence of her early infantile attitudes was revealed in the phantasies underlying the action with her fæces, spoken of above. I have already mentioned that the fæces were to her weapons used in hatred against her parents. This implied that the fæces had dangerous propensities—dangerous for her own body and for her husband's genital about to enter her body, and therefore she had to remove them before intercourse. There were further phantasies in which her fæces stood for her internalized parents attacking her in the same way in which she had attacked them, especially with regard to sexual activities and sexual pleasures. The hold of this compulsive action gradually lessened, and disappeared for long periods, but with recurrence at times of crisis.

(I am not intending here to give the details of the analytic work and the ways in which these many phantasies came to light, as I only wish to show how these infantile impulses and anxieties influenced the development of her character and her behaviour as a grown up woman.)

Her fæces also represented bad dangerous children, and this connected with the hatred she had felt against her mother's pregnancy and the younger brother, but also against her older brothers and sisters.

She could not desire to have children herself, and when she had a child she could not enjoy him; the bad relation to her younger brother with all its anxieties was repeated in the relation to her own child. Hence also the rigid rules which she observed in her dealings with her child; they expressed the fear of her own destructiveness. Fears that her mother would harm the patient's child and thus retaliate for her attacks upon her young brother were shown by the fact that for years she had not allowed her mother near her child, and that in the transference situation she could not imagine coming to see the analyst if she became pregnant. This fear continued for a long time; she was truly convinced that the analyst would attack the child in her womb.

The mother was such an evil figure to her and she was so full of distrust towards her that she could not see any other motive in her mother's obvious attempts to reconcile her with her father, but that of deceit.

Although consciously fond of her husband she did not really trust him. She had used him so much as a tool for making trouble with her parents that he too had become bad, and moreover contemptible. Yet there was fondness for him and for her child and this was for a time the only evidence of the hidden love for her parents and her brothers and sisters which had enabled her to build up whatever constructive elements there were in her relation to people, to marry and become a mother. As the analysis progressed, it appeared that she had so much stifled and repressed

8

her early love feelings, because her excessive hatred and the ensuing anxieties and guilt had made it impossible for her to stand up to the conflict between her love and her hate. She had resorted to seeing herself as a victim of her parents' badness; she had re-inforced any legitimate grievances, and this in turn meant that she was driven to keep the bad, persecuting parents under severe control.

Love had to be altogether denied, both in herself and in others. A favourite conscious image of hers, which she applied to herself, was of "a drop of pitch in the barrel of honey", which ruined the whole. Her *unconscious* phantasy was of a drop of honey in a barrel of pitch; and this pure drop of genuine love and goodness, representing the good breast, the good penis, the good milk, the loving united parents, must never be brought out, drawn upon or used. It was only a drop, whereas the pitch was inexhaustible— the bad fæces, the dead and destroyed persons, the hate and the greed. These must always therefore be brought out and shown and acted upon, since only in this way could the one small drop of goodness be safeguarded. If this were brought out and used, it was lost for ever, and ruined by the bad pitch with which it would then inevitably be mixed up. If love were brought out from its secret hiding place, it could not be kept apart from the terrible hatred, which would swallow it up.

It was ultimately these underlying phantasies which had built up the character traits of hatred, meanness and dependence in this patient, and distorted her sense of external reality, as well as inhibited her pleasure in sexual intercourse and in bearing and suckling her child.

The analysis of these early anxieties, phantasies and defences brought about considerable changes in the patient's personality and life.

At the beginning of the analysis she was already qualified as a social worker, but was doing very poor work, because she could never make use of her intelligence and knowledge, nor of any sympathetic understanding of the people under her care. Her work greatly improved, she became skilled and competent and able to see the psychological factors in the needs of other people.

Her relation to both her parents became much more satisfactory, by no means free from greed, envy and hatred, but without denying her hostility and without justifying it on the grounds of the parents' badness. She made friends with her mother first, although for a long time this was very superficial and largely used for the purpose of controlling her father. But gradually she became able to feel and to admit love and admiration for her father, particularly after her sexual wishes towards him and her frustration in this respect had come out into the open in the analysis. Whilst in the past she had been an adept in bringing out his worst qualities, she now was able to evoke his kind and generous traits. This again interacted with her improved relation to her mother, for, in terms of the Œdipus complex, she could now allow her mother to have a good husband.

She developed a more realistic attitude and saw her parents' faults and weaknesses with a clearer eye, whilst giving up her impossible demand that they should be perfect. Thus she also became less dependent.

An important part of the analysis preceding these changes consisted in the filling out of the gaps in her memories, including memories of early sexual play with her brothers. This brought about a re-valuation of her early experiences, and retrospectively the figures in her early life assumed friendlier, human qualities. Her whole previous relation with her brothers and sisters had been to exploit their faults. Her aim had always been to project her bad feelings, impulses and bodily substances on to the other children, so that the good might be in her. In this phase of the analysis she was for the first time able to think in an objective (sympathetic) way of her parents' feelings, their cares and responsibilities, their anxieties and disappointments in relation to their children, and specifically she was able to think of her father and mother, when one brother risked his life as an airman. She had also become able for some time to perform some real service for her family and to experience a sense of responsibility towards them, whilst at the same time fearing her own aggression less.

She could better face difficult and unpleasant realities in her own daily life, e.g. serious financial trouble.

This result was not brought about without great quantities of hate, fury, and anxiety being experienced in the transference situation which led to very aggressive behaviour towards the analyst. There appeared the phantasies of having inside herself damaged and ruined parents (and brothers and sisters) threatening her with revenge and destruction. The whole of her life and of her relations with her family and the analyst expressed her need to control and keep at bay her internal enemies who would, if they were not controlled, attack and destroy her, physically and mentally. She was particularly afraid of the attacks they would direct against her femininity and her sexual life.

It was the working through of these terrifying phantasies which led to the favourable changes already described. A climax was reached when she arrived at the wish to have another child. She conceived her second child with conscious desire, and this time she could enjoy her motherly functions and was happy in the suckling and tending of the baby. At the same time she had also developed a happier relation with her first child, and became capable of tender feelings towards her family and friends, and of giving active help to them.

4. SUMMARY

I have selected only those aspects from a long and full analysis which illustrate my thesis that the defence of manic control is developed as a means of dealing with overwhelming anxieties.

It leads to faulty ego development, such as malformation of character, impoverishment of feelings and emotions, distortion of the sense of reality which affects the relation to persons, and to a profound inability for enjoyment and happiness. The analysis of the manic defence has to go back to the earliest levels of development, to the earliest pre-verbal phantasies, impulses and anxieties against which this defence was evolved, as well as to work through the elaborations of these patterns in later development and in the patient's actual life. When the patient in the transference situation is gradually brought face to face with the conflicts which his weak ego at the time was unable to cope with, he comes to find better solutions and more adequate defence through the strengthening of his ego which accompanies and is the outcome of the analytic work. This strengthening of the ego is bound up with a diminution of the power of the archaic super-ego—the frightening internalized figures—and the evolution of a more realistic and more mature super-ego.

VIII

CRITERIA FOR INTERPRETATION[1]

(1939)

1. INTRODUCTION

THE question of the criteria by which we test the validity of our convictions in analytical work is one of great practical importance in the day to day carrying on of our work, as we reflect upon the progress and the resistance to progress of our patients. It enters into the discussion of controversial issues between analysts, since everyone who puts forward new contributions may and should expect to be challenged as to the basis of his views and the tests and verifications to which he has subjected them. Lastly it is of central importance in the statement of our theory for the non-analytic public, who have the right to challenge our premises and conclusions and to be shewn our methods of testing and verification.

It is my constant practice in training students of general psychology and child development to emphasize the key significance of method, and to shew that no hypotheses or conclusions can be evaluated except by reference to the methods upon which they are based. This is surely true with regard to analysis also, and not only analytic theory as a whole, but also the many detailed controversial issues in which we are all interested. In the last resort, differences of opinion as to fact and theory largely come down to differences of method, methods of discovery and methods of testing and verification.

2. THE MATERIAL OF OUR WORK

The psychological data upon which we form our judgements as to the patient's unconscious feeling, wish or intention, his forgotten history or repressed knowledge of present events, are not only very extensive but very varied in their nature. It is impossible to do justice to their variety and complexity in a brief summary. In outline they may be grouped as follows:—

[1] *I.J.P.A.*, Vol. XX, Pt. 2. A paper read to the International Congress of Psycho-Analysis, Paris, 1938.

(1) The facts of the patient's behaviour as he enters and leaves the room and while he is on the couch, including every detail of gesture and tone of voice, pace of speech and facial expression, any routine or any changes in behaviour and expression; every sign of affect, or change in affect, its particular nature and intensity, in its associative context.

(2) His free associations, with every detail of content and verbal style, including any obvious omissions as well as what is actually said, and all the emphasis and distortions of emphasis. Special points are the repetition of previously recounted incidents and the affective and associative context in which this occurs; changes occurring in memory material or in the mode of reference to people or to circumstantial facts; idiosyncratic phrases or modes of speech; the patient's selection of facts and details for comment, noting omissions as particularly as inclusions, for example, regarding any real incident which has occurred in the analytic room, in public affairs, or in his own life or family history.

(3) The patient's dreams and waking phantasies, together with all their associations.

(4) His behaviour and attitudes to other people in the outside world, as reported by him or (sometimes) as reported by them or seen by themselves.

I would emphasize how much attention the analyst pays to behaviour in all the details of his work. As analysts we ought not to lend ourselves to the false antithesis between analytic and behaviouristic studies. This antithesis is useful to our critics, but it is false. Freud has taught us to appreciate sequences and connections in behaviour which escape the notice of other people.

3. Our Perception of Unconscious Meaning

As we listen to the associations and note the behaviour and signs of affect of our patients, certain mental processes, partly conscious, partly unconscious, are evoked in ourselves. We may, for example, deliberately recall the end of the last hour as we note his material in the beginning of the present one, or make a deliberate effort to compare what he is saying to-day about a certain person with what he was saying a week or a month ago. On the other hand, memories of what he has said earlier, of the facts we have already gathered, come welling up spontaneously in our minds. We find ourselves evaluating directly, by unconscious processes, his mood, his affect, his attitude to ourselves. If our own minds are working freely so that we are alive and sensitive to the transference situation, not inhibited in our memory and our judgement of the present material or of the patient as a whole, if we can identify ourselves with the patient, with the whole patient, but not too closely or automatically with the particular facet he is presenting at the moment, the meaning of his words and conduct becomes plain to us. Exactly in the same way as the patient's associations to the manifest content of the dream, bringing up new thoughts, new memories, new affect, new phantasies, break down the manifest content into apparently disconnected fragments and then rebuild these into a very different whole of dynamic significance, so does the material of the whole hour, or whole phase of analysis, yield fragments of meaning, of past and present significance which, as the hour or whole period unfolds, gradually form themselves into a new and more deeply significant whole. Sometimes it is a single remark revealing a specific phantasy or memory or attitude of mind, a single comment on a real situation, which gives the meaning to every detail of what has gone before, all the rest of the material then falling into place and becoming an intelligible whole. Sometimes this emergence of meaning is a gradual and cumulative process.

Now this becoming aware of the deeper meaning of the patient's material is sometimes described as an intuition. I prefer to avoid this term because of its mystical connotation. The process of understanding may be largely unconscious, but it is not mystical. It is better described as a *perception*. We perceive the unconscious meaning of the patient's words and conduct as an objective process. Our ability to see it depends, as I have said, on a wealth of processes in ourselves, partly conscious and partly unconscious. But it is an objective perception of what is in the patient, and it is based upon actual data.

In attempting to explain analytical work to non-analytic students, I am accustomed to give them a series of examples, starting from quite obvious ones which only the most inhibited person could fail to appreciate. For instance: a boy of five years of age, one day at a meal, addressing no one in particular, said in a very subdued way, "I don't like dreams: they are horrid things"; and then, after a pause, "and another thing—I don't have any".

Now I find that every hearer, save the most obtuse, appreciates perceptually that in his denial the boy actually makes a positive statement, namely, that his dreams are so horrid that he wishes he did not have any, and cannot bear to remember them. The ordinary hearer does not set out his awareness of this in conceptual terms, as analysts have learnt to do, using it as a means of generalizing the mechanism of denial; but everybody perceives the immediate concrete meaning. From such an example, which the man in the street can read, one may pass step by step to examples of words and behaviour which yield their meaning only to the analysed, and the analytically trained; but there is no essential difference in the process of perceiving the unconscious mind through overt words and conduct, between such simple instances and those we deal with in the analytic hour. The difference lies in the degree of education. By his own analysis and his cumulative experience of others, the analyst is trained to perceive meanings which would be obscure to the untrained mind.

Our perceptions become thus trained, partly by direct experience in our own analysis and in listening to others. We come to understand the various mechanisms of the mental life by living through them in ourselves and with our patients. But in part this education is conceptual, since we bring to bear upon our concrete material a wider knowledge drawn from more general studies, such as the facts of the overt sexual life among children and adults, the direct observation outside analysis of the talk and conduct of young children, and the systematized knowledge of their successive phases of development. If such knowledge has been well and truly assimilated, it works implicitly in our perception, in just the same way as his knowledge of the habits and plumage and distribution of birds is implicit in the perception of the ornithologist when he looks at a new migrant on a spring day. But at any moment in our work we may deliberately call up, in a systematic way, our knowledge of what people or children do at different ages, in reality or in phantasy, or the comparative facts of the sexual life, in order to judge whether some experience is likely to be a true or only a phantasied piece of history.

4. THE TESTING AND VERIFICATION OF OUR PERCEPTIONS

I have claimed that our awareness of unconscious meaning in analytic work is of the nature of a perception; a perception rather

than an inference. Yet like an inference it can and does receive
confirmation or correction in many different ways.

Let us begin by considering what happens if our interpretation
is *incorrect*.

As we know, interpretations can be incorrect in two ways: they
can be (*a*) false, and (*b*) incomplete.

Unless we are the veriest tyros or "wild" analysts, it is not very
easy to make an interpretation that is completely false; it may
happen to the beginner. If what we say bears *no* relation to the
truth of what is in the patient's mind, it leaves him cold. Doubtless if we went on making statements that were completely untrue,
the patient would begin to do something about it. If we did behave
in this way, it is certain that we should be revealing signs of
affect in ourselves, either of doubt and confusion or of an obtuse
and pontifical pseudo-certainty; and to these signs of affect in us,
the patient would undoubtedly react. His anxieties and disappointments would cause him to leave us and not return. That
is to say, he would respond appropriately to the affective state
in the analyst's mind which led to this stupidity or uncertainty
or untruth. Such a situation would certainly mean that we had
not listened to what the patient had said; it must be rare among
trained analysts.

Far more common, occurring indeed from time to time in the
experience of every one of us, is an interpretation which is false by
its selection or by its emphasis; by being incomplete or by weight-
ing too heavily one aspect of the truth to the detriment of another.
We know that such incomplete or falsely emphasized interpretations may stir up the strongest responses in the patient. Signs of
acute or unmanageable anxiety of one form or another appear,
according to the patient and the specific nature of our error. The
anxiety may be of such a form and degree as to hold up the
analysis altogether, or to risk its breaking off. We are accustomed
to read these responses as a sign that our words have expressed
either a half or a distorted truth, and need addition or correction.
If we can then bear to know our own limitations and to listen
objectively to the words and ways in which the patient then
expresses his anxiety, he will often shew us where our error lies
and the specific nature of our mistake.

Each patient has his own way of doing this. One of my own, a
woman, if I should miss an essential theme in the transference
situation during one hour's analysis, or place the wrong emphasis

upon one part of it, invariably brings me the missing or the under-emphasized theme the next day, fully worked out and elaborated *in relation to her husband*—either having been acted upon in the meantime, or merely felt. This happens in the clearest possible way; so much so that if at the end of an hour I become aware of such a mistake in my interpretation, but too late to rectify it, I can predict with certainty the character of her relation with her husband during the interval, and the nature of her associations at the beginning of the next hour. Such a mechanism gives one a very strong motive for avoiding these temporary errors, since they disturb the patient's external life so much; but it provides an excellent test of the truth of one's interpretations.

Other patients have other ways of doing the same thing for us—provided only that they have a general trust in our understanding.

To consider now *correct interpretations:* and to discuss, first,

A. Interpretations regarding the *present*, whether unconscious feeling, phantasy or intention, or external situation: We get our confirmations and proofs in the following among other ways:

(1) With preconscious interpretations, or those concerning external facts, the patient may give verbal assent. A child may actually say, "Yes, how did you know—did someone tell you?" Or, "How did you know—do ideas like that come into your head?"

(2) Interpretations of unconscious trends may lead these to become conscious, if not at once, then after a time. Whereas the trend had previously been merely implicit in associations or in behaviour, there may now be conscious elaboration of images and the meaning of images, with conscious co-operation and appropriate affect.

(3) There may be further associations which from their specific nature confirm our view, either by amplifying the unconscious attitude or phantasy which was interpreted, or by linking it with external situations in the patient's relation to us or to other people.

(4) There may be a change of associations and of attitude such as we should expect, given what we already know of the patient's general modes of response, and of his specific mode of response to our knowing specific things about him. E.g. there may be a conscious repudiation, in such terms as to provide a confirmation, if it expresses guilt and terror such as would be felt and only felt if our previous interpretation had been correct.

(5) The patient may on the following day bring a dream which carries on and elaborates and make much plainer the unconscious phantasy or intention which had been interpreted. Not only so, but he may recount a dream immediately upon our interpretation, one which he had not told us up to that point, but which had already been partially analysed before being told, some of its essential meaning having been expressed in the patient's behaviour on the couch or in his other associations, the relief of anxiety connected with this part of the latent content of the dream lifting the repression of the dream itself.

(6) Memories of past real experience may be recovered as a result of interpreting present unconscious trends, memories which link these trends to real experiences and make both intelligible.

(7) Inferences as to external situations which had previously been rejected by the patient may be admitted, or voluntarily brought up by the patient, after the interpretation of unconscious feelings or phantasies, these now being seen as responsible for the denial.

(8) One of the most important tests of the correctness of our specific interpretations is the resulting diminution in specific anxieties. This may be shown in a number of different ways. E.g. there may be bodily signs of relief from anxiety, such as relaxing of rigid muscles, stilling of restless or stereotyped movements, change in tone of voice. With a child we can see relief in his facial expression, voice, movement and bodily poise, as well as in the ensuing changes in his play, which becomes richer, freer and more varied.

(9) The resolution of anxiety is seen also in the patient's associations, which may show that the whole unconscious phantasy situation has been changed, with new material emerging as a result of the right interpretation. It is not, however, a matter of the mere lessening in amount of anxiety, but also of a change in its direction. New problems are opened up, with new anxieties, connected in specific ways with those just now interpreted. We learn to look for these specific connections, and to use them as a test of our interpretations. For instance, when phantasies elaborating the persecuting mother imago have been interpreted, and this anxiety is lessened, the patient may then be more able to take up a feminine position, identifying himself with his mother, both in phantasy and in memories; but this in its turn will bring up the

anxieties connected with the sexual and aggressive aspects of the dangerous father imago; the analysis of these will bring then further relief, and change the internal situation once more, in a connected way.

(10) These changes in amount and direction of anxiety have their greatest significance in the transference situation. It is what happens in the transference situation, indeed, which provides us with an acid test of the correctness of our perceptions. A valid interpretation may change the phantasy picture of the analyst from a dangerous to a helpful figure. In the case of a child, the room may have seemed to be full of terrible roaring lions; and when the meaning of this phantasy in reference to the child's dread of the analyst is interpreted, the lions become kind and friendly ones. Yet a valid interpretation will not inhibit the further development of phantasy, in the way in which mere reassurance will do. If interpretation has been both true and adequate, phantasies will unfold more richly, and memories stir more freely, whether in the play of the child or the words of the adult.

(11) We can often thus in many ways predict the course of the analysis, both its general course and its detailed immediate future. Such predictions, whether or not expressed, may be fulfilled in a manner that is both dramatic and of great scientific value, as testifying to the validity of our perceptions and conclusions, i.e. of our interpretations.

So much for our interpretations regarding present unconscious trends or real events.

B. Now to discuss our reconstructions of the patient's *past history and past feelings*.

We are led to infer such and such happenings in the past, by bringing together what is already known about his experiences with what he is showing us here and now of his attitudes and feelings and behaviour to people in the present; and above all by his unconscious or preconscious attitudes to ourself as his analyst. A common source of evidence is the repetition of some early relation which has not yet been recovered in memory. The details of his behaviour on the couch, with all its affective colouring, often enable us not merely to infer that such and such happened, but that it happened at about such and such an age, since it is so characteristically the behaviour of a child of a given period of life. As a rule, we also have a circumstantial setting into which we can piece our interpretations and which links with our view of the original date of the behaviour now being repeated. The repetition of this piece of behaviour, often with an associated memory in a series of varying contexts, contexts with a certain quality of verisimilitude, enable us to infer a past real experience.

Confirmation of these inferences then comes in various ways: E.g. (*a*) New memories, either not yet told to us or long forgotten by the patient, emerge as a result of our interpretations; (*b*) such memories may directly corroborate what has been inferred, may be new instances of the same kind, or, whilst different, may yet be linked with our inferences, historically or psychologically; (*c*) further associative material may arise which makes intelligible the *forgetting* of this and other experiences, as well as present attitudes; (*d*) corroboration may be gained from outside sources such as friends and relations. Such corroboration from outside is not necessary for the analytic work itself, but it is useful from the scientific point of view, as an additional and independent proof. (*e*) We can correct our impressions of the past history of the patient by referring to our general knowledge of the actual behaviour of human beings at various ages, and the various phases of development, social, intellectual and sexual; having regard not only to general characteristics at different ages, but also to the known range of individual differences.

Finally, in surveying our accumulated individual histories and knowledge of individual mechanisms for the general formulation of psycho-analytic theory, we have regard to such general principles of scientific method as the internal consistency of the various parts of the theory, and the scope and variety of facts which it articulates and makes intelligible.

This is by no means a complete account of our modes of testing and proof, but must serve to indicate their type and range.

5. Psycho-analysis as Scientific Method

Let us now consider the advantages and limitations of psycho-analysis as a scientific method, and its relation to other techniques of research.

It is clear that the relation of the analyst to the patient's mind is not and never can be that of the physicist or the biologist to his material. We are dealing with living minds, in a living relation to ourselves, and cannot stand outside that relation in complete detachment.

Moreover, our material changes from moment to moment. Our

patient's thoughts and feelings and intentions do not stay still while we examine and compare them. The changes occurring are themselves part of our evidence. They not only bring us new data, but are themselves data by which we gain understanding of the patient's history and present life.

It is, however, increasingly recognized that the ideals of the physical sciences do not provide the true criteria of scientific method for the psychologist. This truth is admitted even by those observers and experimenters working in the narrower and more objective fields of the mind, the description of behaviour for its own sake, the laws of learning, the study of remembering and forgetting and imagining on the conscious level. Earlier attempts to force psychological methods into the mould of the physical sciences have proved sterile for the experimentalists. As one of the leading academicians recently pointed out, the experimental psychologist is bound to be as much clinician as experimenter. That is to say, he is obliged to recognize that he is studying the complex responses of a highly developed organism which have been called forth to meet the demands of a very unstable and varying objective environment. But if the environment is violently simplified it is mere superstition to trust that the subject's responses also become simplified in a corresponding manner. They become different, but are just as likely to become yet more complex. "Stability of determination, not simplicity of structure, in objective determining factors, is what we need to make our experiments convincing. Stability of determination is compatible with complexity and even with considerable variation of objective determinants."[1]

In many recent academic studies of psychological phenomena in children and adults, attempts have been made to devise experimental and observational methods which are adequate to the complex and dynamic responses of human beings, without reducing the objective situation to a false and sterile simplicity. Such studies approximate more and more in this respect to the method of the analyst.

If stability of objective conditions be one of the demands which must be met by a scientific technique, how far can psycho-analysis pass this test? It can in one respect, but not in another. We do attempt to maintain a constant situation, one which approximates to the stable objective situation of the experimentalist; and that

[1] F. C. Bartlett, *Nature*, August 31st, 1929.

not merely with regard to the physical setting out of our work, but much more significantly, with regard to the psychological atmosphere. We do our best to keep our own attitude to the patient calm, objective and undisturbed by his words or feelings or behaviour to ourselves or to others. Our own responses to him, our real responses, as distinct from the patient's phantasies and feelings about us, are of a constant nature, with the single-minded purposes of understanding and helping the patient to understand. (Needless to say, I am not claiming infallibility for the analyst; neither he nor the experimentalist attains a perfect technique. I am speaking of the heart of the matter. When we fail, there are reasons for our failure, which it is our business to know about and correct if we can.)

Yet there is an essential and deeply significant difference between our method and that of the mere observer. We do not merely listen and record; we respond. And thereby we alter the situation as we go along. What we have to do for the patient is not to give him an indifferent experimental task which he may forget if he chooses the next moment, and which never has any personal meaning, but to say to him something which may be intensely painful or frightening or humiliating, something which he may have fought all his life not to hear and not to know about himself; our words have the greatest possible dynamic influence and may change the situation almost out of recognition.

Even this does not, however, altogether stultify the scientific demand for constancy and objectivity of condition. We do not seek to effect changes in our patient's mind in the way in which the educator or the priest or the politician does. We do not aim to mould him according to our notions of what he should be like, but only to enable him to make his own changes in himself, by understanding his own deeper wishes and counter-wishes. We are not concerned with our own purposes, but with his. Since we tell him simply what he has shown us of his own feelings or imaginings or intentions or thoughts, aim merely to make conscious his unconscious trends by putting them into words when he cannot do so for himself, we do in fact maintain a constant objective situation of friendly truthfulness, and truthful goodwill. And this constant atmosphere of truth and friendliness and objectivity is absolutely essential to our therapy as well as to our science. It is the only basis upon which the revealing and healing changes in the patient himself can occur. We have thus the strongest possible motives for maintaining it to the best of our abilities.

Another important element of scientific method is the isolation of the factors in any situation so as to get a differential response. Now this aim we cannot achieve in any detailed or deliberate way, being so much more observers than experimenters. And yet in one broad and significant sense, we are doing this all the time. The very constancy of the conditions we create, our own detachment and objectivity, provide an isolation. We tell the patient as little as possible about ourselves, reveal our private lives, our personal aims and values as little as possible, precisely in order to throw his into a high light. The purpose of our actual behaviour to the patient, those aspects of our real selves which do operate towards him, our goodwill, our friendliness, our tolerance, our dispassionate aims, our pursuit of the analytic aim and that alone, themselves further the scientific isolation of the patient's feelings, memories and phantasies, above all of his relation towards ourselves, as repeating and expressing his true unconscious aims towards his parents. In this way we isolate the psychological factors from the circumstantial. In the analytic room, we protect the patient's mind from such intrusive external stimuli, since we have found that it is only in so far as we are able to do this that his deepest secrets will yield themselves up, and the so long buried phantasies and rejected wishes and hidden anxieties raise their heads and come forth into the light of understanding.

Another commonplace of scientific method is the repetition of situations, either by the original or by other investigators, in order that first conclusions may be verified or corrected. Now repetition in the strictest sense we certainly cannot have, since every experience changes the living mind, and every word or look of the analyst affects the patient's feelings and responses towards him. The patient's relation to us is not the same to-day as it was yesterday. We cannot have exactly the same situations over again in order to test and refine our interpretations. This difficulty is, however, not peculiar to psycho-analysis; it pertains to every significant type of psychological research. The mere appearance of experimental repetition was only created by choosing indifferent material and working with adults. No one working with children in any field can imagine that he may have an exactly similar situation to-day and yesterday and to-morrow. Time and growth and emotion are inexorable in their disturbance of the experimental machine.

Repetition does, however, occur in a different way. Every patient brings up the same essential situation time and time again, always with a difference, but with the same general structure— e.g. the same feelings and phantasies of fear or suspicion or defiance or over-compensated love or hate towards ourselves. Some have a way of repeating at successive phases of the analysis their tale of a particular incident in their lives. Such repetitions, part of the stuff of every analysis, give us a chance not only to note the new elements in the situation or story, with changes in affect, but also to confirm or modify our previous conclusions as to its meaning in the patient's history.

One of the essential difficulties of our work from the scientific point of view is that repetition by others with the same patient is impossible. In most other fields of psychology, it is possible to have more than one observer present, so that records and judgements can be compared. In analytic work this is quite out of the question, a serious handicap both for ourselves and for the general public. But we cannot alter this fact, and have to accept it as a limitation for pure science, imposed upon us by the very nature of the human mind.

To set against this very real scientific limitation of our work we can, however, place one of its great advantages, viz.: that the study of any one individual is highly intensive. In no other field of science is the study of one organism, one mind, carried on for such a long period and in such an exhaustive manner. To set against the small number of our patients, we have the enormous mass of material with all the minute inter-relations of data. It is a misleading prejudice in the psychological field, brought from the physical sciences, to assume that number of cases is more important than conditions and detail of observation. If instead of persons we consider actual wealth of data, variety of situations, even mere number of hours of observation, then our work may claim a high quantitative status.

9

IX

A SPECIAL MECHANISM IN A SCHIZOID BOY[1]

(1939)

In his comprehensive paper on "The Theory of Symbolism",[2] Ernest Jones referred to the relation between true symbolism and other forms of indirect representation such as the metaphor. In this connection I wish to offer here a brief description of a special mechanism occurring in the analysis of a schizoid boy of fifteen and a half years of age. I hope to expand this account at some future date, and to go more fully into the various problems of the nature and function of symbolism with which it is obviously linked.[3] In this note I am concerned only incidentally with these more general issues. My purpose is to describe the special mechanism observed, of *the acting out of a metaphor*.

The patient has been in analysis a few months. He has acute hypochondriacal symptoms. His actions are often "queer" and apparently meaningless.

One day he told me that he had been trying to make a parachute out of an old umbrella, and that, if he succeeded, his intention was to take it to the top floor of the house, attach to it a basket containing the cat, of whom he was very fond, and let the basket down from the window by means of the parachute. (He did not succeed, but spent some days on the attempt.)

The meaning of this aim and action became clear only slowly. I will not detail the steps by which we arrived at it, but give its significance as uncovered after about a month of further analysis.

The boy's parents were both of advanced political views, "bohemian" in their sexual morality and general ways of life. They had lived apart for several years and were now divorced. The mother was happily re-married. The boy had been brought

[1] *I.J.P.A.*, Vol. XX, Pts. 3 and 4.
[2] *British Journal of Psychology*, Vol. IX, 1918; reprinted in *Papers on Psycho-Analysis*.
[3] Of relevant literature other than Ernest Jones's paper and the seventh section of Freud's "The Unconscious" (*Collected Papers*, Vol. IV, especially p. 130), I would refer in particular to Melanie Klein, "The Importance of Symbol-Formation in the Development of the Ego", *I.J.P.A.*, Vol. XI, 1930, and to Ella Sharpe, "Psycho-Physical Problems Revealed in Language" (read before the Fifteenth International Psycho-Analytical Congress, Paris, 1938).

up since he was about seven years of age by the mother's sister and parents, of a rigidly Non-conformist religion and provincial morality. The mother had herself rejected all the ways of life of her own parents, and had been loud in her criticism of all her family. She was now wishing to take her son to live with her again, and sought to detach his feelings from his grandparents and his aunt by severe criticism of their views and standards, and of their competence to educate him.

The family had been very devoted to the boy, and in earlier years he had been very attached to them. But his mother's criticism of them and the prospect of going to share her more liberal home had fostered an extreme contempt for the family in general and for his grandmother in particular. The conflict of loyalties was terrible, and made him extremely frightened of those with whom he still lived.

At the time of the parachute incident, his mother was still trying, as she had been for some months and even years, to compel the boy himself to choose between her and his grandmother, throwing upon him the responsibility for leaving the family to whom he owed so much. It became clear that he was incapable of such a choice; and a little later on the mother took upon herself this responsibility for the rejection of the grandparents and fetched the boy to her own home. After a stormy period of re-adjustment, a new phase of life began, in which there was more external satisfaction.

Until she took this decisive step, however, the mother was expecting the boy to reject his grandmother. This was felt by him as a demand that he should "throw her out", and in his intention to put the cat out of the window, but in a basket attached to the parachute, he was dramatizing this demand that he should "throw the grandmother out", but at the same time was trying to "let her down gently". That is to say, in the parachute incident he was *acting out a metaphor*.

Since then, he has acted out, or sometimes expressed in his associations, many other metaphors, such as "giving him a smack in the face", "making him feel small", etc., so that I have learnt to recognize this special mechanism and to decode the metaphor more quickly.[1]

---

[1] In a private communication Dr. Clifford W. Scott has told me that he, too, has found that the behaviour of the schizophrenic is very often to be understood as the acting out of significant words or a metaphor. "It is always a charade, never a play."

Other metaphors are expressed in the boy's hypochondriacal symptoms, such as a blurred vision, which represents the feeling that his parents "cannot see straight". Many others are acted out on the couch by small movements of the fingers, hands or feet. For example, one day he had been making certain graceful pulling movements with his right hand and fingers which I had not yet understood, but having certain other material to go upon in his associations I said that he seemed to be feeling that he was being moved about by other people, his parents and family in the external world, without regard to his own wishes, and that this was connected with his unconscious phantasy that he was being moved about by people stronger than himself inside him. (We had already had plenty of material showing the phantasy of people inside him.) He replied: "Yes, I was just thinking that the movements I was making with my hand now were like those you make when you play with puppets". That is to say, he was feeling himself to be a puppet in the hands of his parents, both his external parents and the phantasied parents in his internal world; and he had to deal with the tremendous anxiety aroused by this situation of complete helplessness against forces within and without himself by the movements of his hand, which reversed the situation and represented him as being in control of other people and them as the puppets.

For some nights previously to his mother's actually taking him away from his grandmother's house, the boy had had attacks of extremely acute anxiety and restlessness, which he tried to deal with by dramatic and not very serious suicidal attempts of various kinds. At one moment when his suggested removal to his mother's was being discussed at home he burst out: "I shall be dead before then". It became clear later on in the analysis that these dramatically staged pictures of a wish to kill himself were from the unconscious point of view representations of his feeling that his grandmother would die if he left her. In metaphorical terms, that she "could not live without him". In unconscious phantasy he was trying to kill her, not himself. The last two nights before leaving his grandmother's, he was quite unable to rest in his own room, but carried his bed first downstairs to the sitting room, and lastly out into the garden: that is to say, he "threw himself out" in a literal bodily way; but unconsciously he was throwing his grandmother out as his mother wished him to do, as well as representing his fear that his grandmother would throw him out because he was siding with his mother against her. He feared, indeed, that he would actually throw himself out of the window in a real attempt at suicide, and wanted to let everyone know this.

In the parachute incident he was trying to let her down gently. This had, however, proved impossible, and so the urgent need had arisen and become stronger and stronger to get rid of the grandmother finally and completely by going to the mother; and yet he could not bring himself to take this step. He represented the urgency of his wish to leave by carrying his bed out of doors, but was incapable of taking the final step until his mother took it for him.

The final step was, for his phantasy, that he and his grandmother would each throw the other out. The external reality of his leaving the grandmother represented the unconscious phantasy of his literally throwing his grandmother out of himself—a sort of vomiting. (There had been many important associations about vomiting earlier, as well as about such things as spilling the plate of porridge and milk which his grandmother had given him, etc.)

And the purpose of this was not only to get rid of the "bad" destroyed grandmother, but also to save the "good" one—to save her from his mother's biting and poisonous words, as well as from his own greed and hatred. The urgency of his need to leave, to throw himself out of the house, also arose in part from his wish to save his grandmother from himself and his mother, to go whilst she was still alive.

When I decode the boy's action or hypochondriacal symptom and put the reconstructed metaphor into words, it always receives his assent and usually the comment "of course". Yet in its acted-out version, the metaphor is free from affect. Feeling is only recovered when the metaphor is stated in words.

The analysis proper, the discovery of the unconscious meaning of the metaphor, alike in its acted-out and its verbal form, has then to begin. We go back to the concrete, literal, sensorial images represented in action; but we now carry with us: (a) their appropriate affect, and (b) their correct object-relations. E.g. the cat stands for the grandmother, the words "throw her out" for his mother's demand that he should throw his grandmother out of his affections. In his unconscious phantasy, his mother poisons his grandmother inside him, and he must vomit her up as a destroyed love object.

His mother's criticism had literally and concretely poisoned the boy's mind against her; in unconscious phantasy, had poisoned the grandmother herself inside him; the urge to throw her out arose primarily from the feeling that she was now inside him, a completely ruined and destroyed object; and he must vomit her up in self-preservation. To throw her out of the window, thus, stood for throwing her out of his own body.

To illustrate the metaphorical significance of the hypochondriacal symptoms: one recurrent trouble is a blurred vision, having no basis in physical reality. The boy feels that he sees everything crooked. He says *he* wants never to have to wear spectacles, but goes on: "Both Daddy and Mummy wear them"; that is to say: "I don't want to be like my parents who 'cannot see straight' ". The external preconscious reference is to their sexual morality, to their having given him full sexual knowledge far too early in his education, with all the intense emotional strain which this brought to him. The unconscious meaning of the metaphor is: "My parents inside me are in a terrible sexual intercourse, in which each destroys the other's genitals"; and ultimately: "I cannot bear them to be in sexual intercourse without wanting to make them hurt and destroy each other. Their intercourse is destructive because it stirs up destructive feelings in me. I don't want them to have intercourse." But we were only able to reach the full meaning of the Œdipus conflict, from the hypochondriacal eye symptom, through the first step of reconstructing the metaphor: "My parents cannot see straight".

As with schizophrenics in general, in this patient words have a far greater conscious significance as things in themselves than with neurotic patients. Words are indeed felt to be far more real than actions. And their affective value cannot be over-rated. With this boy, it is the metaphor *in its verbal form* which is the vehicle of affect.

Early in the analysis, the boy had wished to tell me certain criticisms of a girl of whom he had been extremely fond, but who had become entirely spoilt in his mind, not by anything which he had seen of her, but by his being *told* by another boy of sexual things which he, in turn, had been told that she had done. My patient was, however, completely unable to mention her name to me or to speak of her. He had to ask his father to tell me what he wanted me to know, since his father already knew it; and even then he could only speak of it to me when I myself first used her name and mentioned what I had been told, together with my interpretation of his feelings and phantasies about it. I had to be the one first to have her name in my mouth and criticize her, and his father had to be the one to destroy her in my mind by telling me what he, the boy, had been told about her misdoings. To express criticism of other people to me, e.g. of his parents, is always to this boy literally and concretely to poison my mind against them, to put poison into my mind—and into them, inside my mind.

The bodily experience of hearing or using words (the breath going in or out, the sound going in or out, the movements and sensations) remains for him an integral part of their reality and their meaning. Words are still felt by this boy, thus, to be the actual words of the people who were first heard to use them. Even in consciousness words are never signs, but always actions and events. In unconscious phantasy they are parts of people's bodies, "bits" of those who used them; and they are now inside him.

Words are, moreover, as I have said, the carriers of affect, of his feelings about both internal and external objects. And yet, since they can also be used in the metaphorical sense, they serve as an ego-syntonic agency. They seem to be the patient's only hold upon external reality, the link between the internal and external worlds. I surmise that they can serve this function because they can both come in and out of the body (as breath, as sound). He can hear his own words, as well as those spoken by other people; and they keep their identity whether they are inside or out. They are not changed or destroyed by being taken in or given out, as bodies and bodily substances are. And so they keep things whole. They link together the inside and the outside; and are clung to desperately, as a defence against all the terrifying pre-verbal phantasies connected with oral and anal wishes and experiences, in which all loved objects are poisoned or bitten up.

In the metaphor, the boy comes as near as it is possible for him to come to reflective or abstract adjectival judgements about people—himself or his parents. Yet the metaphor cannot be retained as such. It carries too much affect, too intense a conflict of feeling. Hence it is constantly being broken down into its concrete sensorial elements (expressed in meaningless actions, hypochondriacal symptoms, vomiting, defæcating, etc.), divorced from their affects and from their object-relationships. And words are treated as having no meaning but their bodily existence. In his symptoms the boy loses relation to external reality, and concerns himself entirely with his internal reality, with his internal objects and their relations to each other—ultimately, of course, with his sexual parents in the Œdipus conflict *inside him*.

In his acting out of the metaphor, the patient is able to deny all feeling and all *meaning*, whether of his actions or of the words with which he so much occupies himself. Words and actions alike are by their divorce degraded to mere bodily experiences. Only by bringing words and actions together can the life and meaning of each be restored.

Much of the work of this patient's analysis, thus, proceeds by first reconstructing the metaphor expressed in his behaviour or his symptoms, and so recovering the affect and relation to external reality. This decoding of the acted-out metaphor is an essential step towards the uncovering of the full unconscious symbolism.

X

TEMPER TANTRUMS IN EARLY CHILDHOOD IN THEIR RELATION TO INTERNAL OBJECTS[1]

(1940)

IN this paper I wish to discuss the phantasies and special mechanisms involved in "temper tantrums", those manifestations of acute anxiety so often seen in children between one and five years. In these outbreaks, children are liable to scream violently, kick, stamp, hit and bite other people, hold their breath, stiffen the body, throw themselves on the floor, and struggle against all control. At the height of the attack the child appears to be deaf to the voice of reason, persuasion or command, and almost inaccessible to external influence.

It is very rarely that such attacks occur in a violent form in the actual work of child analysis, since we can usually read the signs of mounting anxiety and anticipate the worst by interpretation. But it is often possible to discern the particular phantasies which without interpretation would lead to tantrums, and to relate the analytic situation in these respects to the circumstances which actually provoke the tantrums, in the child's external life, as well as to his earlier experiences.

During the last few years, I have analysed several children who throw light on these phenomena, and have also had an adult patient whose behaviour on the couch at moments of extreme anxiety was extraordinarily like that of a child in a violent tantrum.

Objective studies of the frequency and distribution of tantrums have shown that they reach a high peak during the second year of life; they then gradually lessen in frequency until the sixth or seventh year, when they become comparatively rare in normal children. They appear to be a phenomenon of normal development, since they occur to some degree with all classes of children in all sorts of general circumstances, although some children in

[1] *I.J.P.A.*, Vol. XXI, Pt. 3. A paper read to the International Congress of Psycho-Analysis, Paris, 1938.

some circumstances are much more liable to such outbursts than others.

The immediate causes of such outbursts are very varied, but a study of all types of provoking situation seems to suggest one common element, viz., that the tantrum is a response to compulsion. Tantrums occur when children are told to do something they do not wish to do, are denied something they wish to have, or when there is some change in the routine of their daily life. Within the ordinary routine they may violently object to being dressed or undressed, being washed or lifted out of the bath, being made to clean their teeth, to put on some clothing they dislike, to go to the toilet, being given an enema; being kept waiting for something they are expecting to receive or to happen, having their bodily movements restricted, being forced to share their possessions with someone else or unable to get hold of someone else's property; being unable to make their wishes understood, being shut out of the activities of other children or the attention of the grown-ups. Tantrums may also occur when the child fails to achieve something he is trying to do, e.g. when he cannot successfully manipulate some physical object. The child's response when this happens shows that he feels this neutral physical object to be defying and attacking him, and defeating his aims, as if it were another human being.

Examples of the provoking situations could be multiplied, and many specific motives can be discerned. In some of these situations, the child's libidinal aims are frustrated. In others, his sublimated sexual wishes and reparation tendencies are defeated. In others again, he shows his castration anxieties and his fear of other people's aggression. But the general character of all the moments which cause this unmanageable anxiety is the *compulsion* exerted upon the child, to do, to have or to endure what he does not want; to lose, or to refrain from doing or being what he does want. The child feels he is up against some force which he cannot control or alter, a person who will defeat all his wishes, rob him of all pleasure, restrict all his movements and reduce him to complete helplessness. He is in the hands of his persecutors.

The violence of the child's struggle in his tantrums is usually so much out of proportion to the actual loss or compulsion that we are obliged to recognize that the most primitive phantasies and anxieties are at work. He is fighting a phantasy mother, rather than the real one with whom he actually struggles. The real denial or command acts like a hair trigger releasing in full force the most primitive persecutory phantasies. If he does not get *this* sweet, his mother is going to starve him. If she puts *this* particular garment upon him, or will not let him get down from her knee at *this* moment, she is going to bind him and reduce him to permanent and complete helplessness. If she insists upon his urinating or defæcating *now*, she is going to castrate him and tear out all his inside. If he cannot build a tower *now*, when he wants to do so, he never will be clever enough to balance one brick on top of another. If he has to give up his toy to a playmate, he never will get it again, or any other toy in the world. Above all, he feels that if he cannot control people and things completely and make them do what he wishes here and now, he himself will be reduced to a complete and helpless loss of everything that he needs and longs for.

The detailed study in analysis enables us to take a further step and to recognize that these phantasied persecutors with whom the child struggles are primarily felt to be inside his own mind and his own body. He projects these internal persecutors upon external thwarting persons, since outside enemies *can* be fought and resisted. To appreciate this helps us to understand the violence of some of the bodily symptoms, such as the bodily rigidity, the kicking and hitting, the momentary deafness and blindness of the child. He is so much alive to the danger inside his body that he becomes for the time being deaf and blind to external reality.

The general theory of internal objects, derived first of all from the work of Freud and Abraham, has now been clearly developed in the various contributions of Melanie Klein and other members of the English group. This paper is concerned not with the elucidation of the general theory of internal objects, but with the way in which an understanding of the various phantasies connected with internal objects serves to illuminate the phenomena of temper tantrums and helps in their analytic treatment.

I will now quote from two cases some material illustrating certain of the detailed phantasies involved in children's tantrums, first from a boy of three and a half and then from an adult obsessional patient.

The boy of three and a half came for treatment because of a particular symptom. His relation with other children in the nursery school was friendly but distant. Every now and then, however, he would separate himself from the others and stand

alone for ten minutes or longer, psychically quite withdrawn, and
with marked tension and spasmodic quivering of his body. These
moments had alarmed his nursery school teacher by their look
of abnormality.

At home, he had from the end of his first year been subject to
specially violent tantrums. I realized during his analysis that
these queer moments of silent withdrawal and tension in the
nursery school were substituted for the tantrums. He was too
frightened of the many other children there to show his fear and
aggression openly.

In the analysis, it soon became clear that the boy's brother, just
one year younger, and their inter-relations with their mother,
provided the dominant factor in his life.

Now from the beginning of his analysis, my patient showed an
absorbing interest in the insides of things, drawers, cupboards,
boxes, the gas fire, electric fire, etc. For instance, he found he
could lift off a portion of the front of the gas fire, and look at its
inside parts. He was always very anxious and eager about this,
wanting to know what they were, to touch them and take them
out; one day he pointed to what he called "the crack", across the
head of a large screw inside this part of the fire, saying: "I don't
like that". Here we obviously have his fear of castration, dread
that he will have a "crack" instead of a penis. But he is quite as
much preoccupied with the fact that this "crack" is *inside*, and
thus shows his fear of a broken and damaged penis, inside himself.

I would emphasize here that in all our interpretation of the
child's play, the place where he puts objects or takes them from
is quite as important as the particular object he is using. The
spatial context of his play will tell us as much as the details of what
he does. He will show us quite clearly, if we look, whether at any
one time he is concerned with internal or external reality, and
with the inside or the outside of his body.

Quite early in the analysis he drew me a picture of his brother.
The drawing showed a little figure in the centre of the page,
encircled by a line going round and round him several times. This
represented the brother inside himself, and being controlled by
him.

His concern with things inside always came out very plainly
after he had, either in reality or in dramatic play, eaten something
he wanted. For example, he found one day in a cupboard a
pencil sharpener which had been left there accidentally by a

previous patient. He said urgently: "Whose is that? I am going to have it". When I told him I could not let him have it as it belonged to someone else, he said: "I *shall* have it, I shall eat it up", and actually pretended to eat it. Then he put it into his trousers pocket and threatened to go away with it. The following day he was anxious and much pre-occupied with everything which might or did contain cut- or broken-up bits, or messy stuff. On another occasion, I was wearing a flowered silk frock with chains of coloured daisies all over it. The boy eyed the dress up and down, but said nothing about it. He took up the plasticine and asked me to cut a large piece into a. number of small pieces. He then stuck all these pieces together, and asked me to roll it all into a ball. Then he said: "Where's the sugar?" (He has a little granulated sugar every morning for cooking play.) He ate all this up. Then he took the large ball of plasticine again and asked me to cut very small pieces off it and roll them into little balls. He was very pleased with these and made me count them. I had to make sixty or seventy. Seeing him look again at my frock, I knew that these many small balls represented the many daisies on my frock, which in turn stood for the children inside me, and that he wanted them. He confirmed this, saying: "I *shall* have that frock and wear it", and tried to mess it up with plasticine. The next thing was to say: "I want you to pull me", that is, to pull him about the floor by means of a skipping rope, he holding one end and I the other. He got me to pull him across the floor, as he lay, three or four times in different positions, sitting down, lying on one side, lying on his stomach. Before he left, I had to make more tiny balls, until all the plasticine was used up, wrap these in a piece of paper and seal the parcel down. He took this parcel home.

On a later day, when much work had been done about his fear of his brother's envy, his guilt about his own greedy wishes to have his father's penis and not to let the brother have it, or to get both the brother's and his own, and thus have a bigger and better one, he repeated this skipping rope play. Again he held one end of it, and I had to hold the other and pull him about as before, dragging him helplessly along the floor in different positions. But now I saw a specific point. The rope had two long wooden handles; one of these was broken, and I always had to hold the broken end while he held the good one. That is to say, I had a bad broken penis, a short one, I was castrated, while he had a long, good, whole one. But in pulling him about I was the more powerful.

What is the meaning of this play with the rope, in which the child gets himself pulled about helplessly in different positions? The first point to be noted is that it always occurred in an oral setting. On each occasion, the boy had been showing me in the clearest way that he wanted to eat up any good thing that he desired—e.g. my frock, or the daisies on it, representing myself as his mother, my breast and the babies and penises I had inside me. He wanted to get these and to eat them up so as to have and keep them for himself.

In his helplessness, allowing me to pull him about over and over again, he was also expressing strong masochistic tendencies.[1] In making me the more powerful person, in spite of the fact that I held the broken handle, the short penis, he was taking the feminine position, while I, in standing up and doing the actual pulling, was in the masculine position. Yet to say that this expressed his masochistic feminine tendencies does not go far enough, since it does not explain the connection of this behaviour or these tendencies with their oral setting. It is after he has eaten the mother and her baby that he stages the rope play, and represents himself as a completely helpless creature. The boy's masochism was thus a way of dealing with his feeling of complete helplessness against his own id, against his oral greed and the intensity of all his desires. Moreover, since he makes me pull him towards myself across the room, he is representing his feeling that the object of his desires is identified with his desires. It is *his mother* who attracts or pulls or drags him towards *her*, who stirs up his greedy desires, who renders him unable to stop wanting her and eating her up. I (his mother) had become identified with his id, his bad, greedy self, because by having a flowered dress, or sugar to eat, or good breasts, a baby inside me, or by being a loving person, I had aroused in him these irresistible greedy destructive impulses.

Moreover, in making me drag him towards me he was representing his phantasy of my eating him up in retaliation, thus

---

[1] I am indebted to my critics in the discussion following this paper at a meeting of the British Psycho-Analytical Society for pointing out to me that the way in which the paper as read presented my interpretations of the child's behaviour was not adequate. It was far too condensed and not well balanced, taking for granted many points that needed further explication in order to show their connections. I have now tried to rectify these omissions.

externalizing his persecution dread, his fear of the bad breast biting him, as he had bitten it, his fear of his brother's vengeful fury as well as of the retaliating mother, retaliating for what he wanted to do to the baby inside her. By letting me pull him towards me with the rope over and over again he not only externalized this dread of persecution, but reassured himself against it. He did not lose me or get eaten up or castrated. I could pull him towards me but did not injure him.

In this way he was also representing me as his super-ego. I had to do the guiding and controlling to keep him safe, and he proved over and over again that I would do so. At one and the same time he said in this play that it was my fault that he was so helpless, and that I must take care of him and be responsible for his safety as well as for him. In this way I stood both for his id and for his super-ego.

Finally, in this masochistic play he dealt with the internal situation of his ego in its helplessness against both his id and his super-ego. He externalized this feeling of helplessness and turned it into a pleasure, libidinizing it through bodily sensations. In other words he was proving himself in full control, able to get pleasure for himself, by staging the play, even though the nature of the play itself was so helpless and masochistic. He really controlled me and his internal situation at one and the same time. Masochistic tendencies in which anxiety situations are sexualized are themselves but one variety of the manic defence.

Now the boy's actual behaviour with his brother in his external life at home showed how strong was his defensive need to control the brother's acts and wishes all the time. If the younger boy was asked whether he would have anything, the elder answered for him: "Yes, Rob will do so-and-so", "No, Rob doesn't want so-and-so". Partly as a result of this the younger child at three years of age did not talk yet, although he was certainly intelligent The elder answered for him in every situation. This answering for the little brother had itself a complex significance. On the one hand he was saying: "My brother *can* talk, listen to him". That is to say, his speaking for the brother was restorative, giving him speech magically, much better speech than he could have had naturally. The elder boy was thus also acting as a super-ego for the little brother, saying that he must talk properly or not at all. On the other hand, he also prevented the little brother from speaking, thus showing his own hatred and wish to castrate the brother, as well as the intensity of his own need to control the younger boy. He had to control him in this way because of his terrible fear of what the younger brother, both actual and internalized, would do if he became bigger, stronger, able to talk, able to do for himself. He would indeed be a persecutor, and must therefore be controlled, kept inside, kept a baby, and castrated all the time. But of course this purpose in its turn increased the elder child's anxiety, since in his mind it gave the brother further motive for revenge.

In his play, the boy thus showed me that his tantrums were not simply due to conflict of feeling in external relationship with his actual brother, or myself as an external person. His mind was dominated by dread of the castrated and vengeful brother felt to be inside himself. His compulsive wetting and dirtying was connected with the phantasy of his brother's cutting, biting, burning and poisoning him inside, in revenge for his own aggressive wishes. His castrated dirty baby brother, who could not talk but only scream, made *him* dirty, cut *him* to bits, made *him* scream, from the inside. He had to defæcate and to scream for two.

The boy gave me another vivid representation of the anxiety connected with his various internal objects. One day he brought his nurse's umbrella to the play-room. He opened it and several times made me twirl it round and round, with the point resting on the floor. When it was going round very fast he named the various spokes, touching them in turn and saying: "That's Nanny, that's Ida, that's May, that's Mummy, that's Daddy, that's Rob"; in other words, they stood for all the people he was afraid of, moving round inside him. The expression of his face as he told me this showed that the whirling umbrella represented his own feeling of everything whirling round outside him, and the blurring of people's faces outside him, under the stress of anxiety, as well as of the sense of their controlling him from the inside. This was connected with his compulsive wetting, since just before he had made a big wet mess on the floor, followed by a half-hearted attempt to wipe it up, which failed.

In the analysis, every aspect of the actual relation of the two brothers had of course to be explored. For example, as both brothers went to the same nursery school at the same time, and my patient's coming for the analysis without his younger brother was the first major separation of the two, his guilt about this wish-fulfilment of his rivalry with his brother was enormous. Everything which he had to play with, I, as his brother, must have also. He was unable to believe that if he had a ball, a pencil, a cup, and there was not a second one for me, I was not burnt up with fury and envy and ready to burn him or bite him to pieces. He dealt with this terror in various ways, but only slowly, as the analysis of his persecution phantasies reduced his anxieties, could we reach any direct expression of his wish to have everything for himself.

He showed his fear of his little brother's wish to castrate him, if he himself became a big boy, got the father's penis, in many ways. As one example, he asked me to model a fire engine with plasticine. When I did so, he gibed at it, saying it "looked funny", it "looked like a horse", or "a donkey"—in other words, I could not do things any better than his little brother. He then said I must put a ladder on the fire engine, but as I began to do so, he said: "I can do it; I can do it better", and quickly modelled a ladder and fixed it on, saying "Aren't I clever?" But immediately, he took his own scissors and cut his own ladder in two, thus anticipating my jealousy for his being clever, and my revenge on him for his scorn of me, that is to say, his brother's revenge on him for having a bigger and better penis. He felt certain I would cut the ladder out of envy, and forestalled me by doing it himself, thus depriving me of the satisfaction; in this way, he also reassured himself against his dread of being assaulted inside.

When he had been in analysis for two months, there came a phase in which he begged me to let him bring his little brother too to the analysis, and his nurse had difficulty in getting him to come alone. This urgent wish arose partly from his fear of his brother's jealousy and anger, partly from brotherly love and reparation wishes. In his mind, if he got good things for himself, grew big, learned to talk, to dress himself and keep himself clean, to jump and play ball, to draw and write, his brother would get smaller, more clumsy and more dirty, never able to talk at all. In his phantasy, there was only one good penis, and if he had it, his brother lost it, was castrated by him. He told me anxiously one day that he wore pyjamas, but his brother wore only nighties.

The boy had had a happy first year of babyhood, with a devoted nurse, who was sent away when the second child was born, two days before my patient's first birthday. The loss of this loved nurse, as a result of the birth of his rival, was the primary stimulus to

his tremendous anxieties.   From then onwards, his temper
tantrums, together with excessive wetting and dirtying of his
garments and his bed, had been extremely acute.

It was mainly because these catastrophic events, the loss of his
nurse, owing to the birth of his deadly rival, came at an age when
oral and anal impulses and the introjection-projection mechanisms
were dominant, that they fostered the boy's phantasies of persecution by his internal objects. The baby brother drove away his
nurse; he took her place, came instead of her. The loss of the
actual good nurse evoked the feeling of loss of the good internalized object, and the hatred and fear of the crying, dirtying
baby stirred up the dread of a bad internal persecutor.

During the analysis, the details of these persecution phantasies
were linked at every point with the real characteristics of the
actual brother and of my patient's real behaviour to him.

To turn now to the adult patient; with him any occasion of
specially acute anxiety in the analytic situation led to behaviour
extraordinarily like severe temper tantrums in a young child. The
patient would shout obscenities or prayers in an extremely loud
screaming voice, and would twist his body, make violent movements, clamp his jaw so tightly that I could hear the teeth grind-
ing; and at times he struck his own forehead violently in a way
that was most painful to watch. The head knocking disappeared
after three years' analysis, but the shouting, although lessened in
frequency and intensity, remained as a sporadic transference
symptom to the end.

(The patient had been diagnosed as a severe obsessional
neurotic, but his paranoia was very acute and the onset of his
illness at twenty years of age had shown a brief catatonic phase.
His mother was an epileptic, and the patient always feared that
he was or would become so himself, although he was not in fact.)

These symptoms on the couch repeated the patient's temper
tantrums of childhood, but in his phantasy they were also a
repetition of the mother's epileptic fits.   His earliest conscious
memory was of seeing his mother, when he was three-and-a-half,
fall down and injure her head in a fit, at a time when she was
pregnant with a child who died at six months of age. He had
certainly heard his mother's cries and groans and thumpings
in her fits at night, as well as in the day, the fits thus being very
closely associated in his mind with parental intercourse.

Now there were many different meanings to this violence on the couch. It represented feelings and phantasies at different levels of the psyche, as well as various real experiences. These could be briefly summarized as follows:—

(1) By his shouting the patient showed his wish to control and defy the analyst as a real person in her own right, in many different ways. He drowned my voice, and told all the world what a dreadful person I was. Because of his fear of rivals, his wife, his friends, other patients, he denied that he was getting any good from me or had any positive wishes towards me. Again, he had to shout in order to let other people know how dangerous he was, and to make sure they would come and save me from him, when he feared his own aggression towards me or his own sexual wishes, which were connected with the most terrific sadistic phantasies. He shouted also in order to make me stop the analysis when it seemed to stir up too strong libidinal and sadistic wishes. He was also in his shouting testing me and the clinic, to see how much we could stand, how indulgent or how frightened we were, how much we could control him. Moreover, his shouting prevented my hearing the mocking laughter which was going on in his mind all the time. This laughter was partly a sexual pleasure at my forcing his thoughts (his fæces) out of him; partly a mocking laughter of defiance, pride and pleasure in foiling me, defying me, putting fæces upon me, etc.

(2) The shouting expressed also a manic control of me as standing for his own actual parents in the Œdipus situation. He was representing the noise of parental intercourse, connected with his real experiences of his mother's cries in her fits in the night. Alternatively, he was stopping parental intercourse; and actually killing his parents in the sexual act. He often brought out a phantasy of being Samson pulling down the house, and feeling that he would willingly kill himself if his death would put a stop to parental intercourse. This wish arose in part from direct Œdipus frustration, partly from his notion that sexual intercourse had actually caused his mother's epilepsy.

(3) His shouting also represented the attack and defence of part objects by part objects. His enormous voice represented a penetrating penis which he was forcing into me in the most sadistic way, as well as hard, forcing fæces, which he forced into me in order to prevent me from getting his fæces—equivalent to his secret thoughts and feelings—out of him.

(4) He was also re-enacting many dramatic early experiences,

assuming now this, now the other part, with the analyst in the corresponding rôle. E.g. his mother had been an over-indulgent weak woman, who stirred up by her indulgence the most awful dread of his severe and tyrannical father. He shouted at me in order to make me hate him and turn him out instead of indulging him. At other times he was acting the part of the mother, shouting in her rage and jealousy of his father, as well as representing her fits. At still other times, he acted the part of his baby brother who had died when he was about four, died "fighting for his life", as his father had described it, in acute bronchitis. The patient was thus fighting me for his life, as well as bringing the baby brother to life again by acting his part. At still other times, he represented himself as the shouting, school-master father, who could control a hundred boys and make them instantly obedient to his will by his tyrannical loud voice.

(5) Yet none of these repetitions of actual people and relations in his external history or of his present relations to me as an external real person brought the most significant key to his tantrums at their worst intensity. The times when his behaviour on the couch came the nearest to that of the screaming, struggling child in an extremity of anxiety were when he was "fighting for his life" *with internal objects*. Internal objects were very plain in the phantasies of this patient. He would, e.g., sometimes apostrophize his own fæces, the hard turd, which was at one and the same time a source of immense pride to him and of the utmost dread, as being a phantasied, cutting, tormenting penis. When, as often, he had difficulty in bringing out such a turd, he would speak to it and say: "Come out, you bugger! I will wring your neck for you!" And in the most violent moments on the couch, when he would strike his own head till the room resounded, he was fighting with the utmost extremity of terror the terrible persecutors within, the epileptic mother, raging in her fits or screaming at the father in her jealousy, the shouting, school-master father, or sometimes the two parents together in the most dreadful sadistic intercourse, as well as at other times the dying baby brother in his struggles for breath. All these, as well as the sadistically conceived part objects, were incorporated and were now in deadly conflict within the patient himself.

(6) Finally, in the shouting and violent movements, the patient was also denying his own inside feelings of love, grief and remorse, with accompanying depression and terror of death. Indeed, one of

the most profound meanings of the shouting and the violent movement was the need to deny the silence of death, the silence of the baby brother after he had died. In this patient's mind the terror of his persecutors was so great that to be good was to be absolutely still, like his mother in her quiet moments after her fits, or the stillness of the baby brother after he gave up fighting for his life and was dead. To be good meant to give up life, to give it to the baby brother and the mother. The violent movements and shouting were therefore the most forcible denial of the necessity which his love and remorse and conscience forced upon him, to give up his life, to be castrated, to lie still and to be subjected to the most terrible attacks of every kind which I, as then representing the tyrant father, the epileptic mother and the brother who died because of the patient's jealousy, would wreak upon him. The patient often told me that to be analysed was to be a wax cat chased through hell by an asbestos dog. He had to be the asbestos dog in his violent movements and shouting, so that I should not turn him into the wax cat who would be altogether melted and destroyed.

It was the interpretation of these terrible internal persecutors which provided the key to the analysis of this patient, gradually relieved the most acute of his paranoic phantasies, caused the convulsive movements and shouting to disappear, strengthened his relations with his external objects and his real present-day environment, recovered his memories and released the long buried feelings of love and grief and remorse towards his parents and the baby brother, and of hope in his present life.

Now in this particular case, there was a very special factor, the influence of the mother's epilepsy. This was certainly the chief reason for the occurrence of these violent tantrums in adult life, as well as for the neurosis as a whole. But the patient's experience of his mother's epilepsy does not nullify the relevance of his case to my general thesis regarding the main significance of tantrums in childhood, since, to his mind, his mother's fits *were* temper tantrums. He saw his mother reduced (by his own jealousy, greed and aggression) to a dirty, kicking, biting, screaming infant, behaving exactly as he felt in his own moments of fear, frustration and fury.

This was in fact to my mind one of the most interesting and illuminating aspects of this case, namely the discovery of what such a terrible experience as seeing one's own mother in epileptic fits can mean to the infant mind. The reality of his mother's epilepsy was appreciated by him in terms (*a*) of his own actual experience of kicking, biting, screaming, dirtying, etc., (*b*) of his own awareness of his intense feelings of annoyance, frustration and rage, together with (*c*) his phantasies of what happens to one's mother if one behaves in this way to her. She, having been subjected to one's own attacks, becomes a dirtying, screaming infant herself. She is poisoned, bitten, made helpless, filled with bad feelings and a violent, destructive penis, and this terrible reality has been brought about by one's own evil magic.

To return in conclusion to tantrums in general: the analysis of situations evoking tantrums in young children shows that these occur when the child feels himself unable to control "good" objects and his persecutors, internal and external, by the ordinary means of appealing or commanding words and actions.

The need to control the actual persons upon whom the child depends for love and food, or whose actual aggression he fears, is itself one of the motives for eating them up and incorporating them. We incorporate not only to keep and to have what we desire, but also in order to control what we fear, by magical means. I have elsewhere quoted the four-year-old girl who nearly choked herself in swallowing her brother's whistle, and told her nurse: "I didn't like the noise it made, and so hid it in myself".

But the need to control is only augmented by this magical incorporation, since the enemies are now at work in a hidden secret way, inside. And the child attributes every failure of his own ego, in his clumsiness, dirtiness, smallness, lack of speech or fatigue, to the attacks of an incorporated enemy. Hence these faults and failures of his own are liable to provoke the tantrum, no less than denial or compulsion from actual persons, since both kinds of thwarting release an unmanageable dread of internal enemies. In children who are liable to acute tantrums, or in all children at the ages when these are specially liable to occur, minor disappointments, denials and compulsions, stirring feelings of rage and helplessness, are instantly interpreted by the child as a violent attack from his internal enemies.

The child's screaming, struggling and rigidity in the tantrum represent his attacking and being attacked by his enemies within and without, against whom he must call up every resource of body and mind, since his life depends upon his getting them once again under his control.

XI

AN ACUTE PSYCHOTIC ANXIETY OCCURRING
IN A BOY OF FOUR YEARS[1]

(1943)

I WISH to describe and discuss the material which follows because it illustrates clearly the interaction between internal and external situations. During the analysis of this four-year-old boy, certain acute anxieties arose in response to particular external events. These events were reflected in a detailed and dramatic way in the content of the anxieties, and in the various defences to which the patient resorted.

The special anxieties I shall discuss showed themselves about the eighth week of analysis, in response to severe environmental stimuli occurring in the sixth week; they were worked through, in their most acute form, during the following month.

I shall describe the boy's symptoms and the general situation of his life; give a brief outline of the course of his analysis up to the crucial happenings in his external life; describe in some detail the extreme anxiety produced by these events; and then discuss the chief meaning of his symptoms and characteristic defences.

DESCRIPTION OF CASE

The boy, Jack, was brought for analysis because of periodic and severe attacks of rage when he was frustrated, and also a "queer" excitement which came on apart from temper, with no immediately obvious stimulus. Apart from these symptoms, his relatives considered him a fairly healthy and happy child, friendly and uninhibited, not specially aggressive or destructive. In the analysis, however, he soon showed that he often had moods of sadness and unhappiness. He had had pneumonia just before he began analysis.

His father had died of tuberculosis when the boy was less than a year old. His mother had a very difficult time nursing the father. After the father's death, the mother went out to business, and Jack

---

[1] *I.J.P.A.*, Vol. XXIV, Pt. 3, 1943. An expanded version of a paper read to the British Psycho-Analytical Society, 1938.

was brought up by his mother's sister. He and his mother still lived with his aunt and her husband. The boy called this uncle "Daddy" and had on the whole a good relation with him.

About a year before the analysis, the aunt was ill for a time and the child was put into a convent for a month. During the year before he came to me, his mother earned her living in evening work at a cinema, and spent the day at home with the boy. During this period, the tantrums and fits of "queer" excitement had become worse. In later talks with the mother, the seriousness of the tantrums became more apparent. She told me that the head of the kindergarten which Jack attended had advised her never to send him to a boarding school, as his "fits" would make him so disliked by the other boys. The course of the analysis showed that this head teacher was correct in her assessment of the seriousness of the boy's psychological difficulties, in spite of the fact that in some ways he appeared so normal.

The home was lower middle class, in a new residential district. The family had very high standards of behaviour, and was prudish and strict. Jack's mother was very particular about manners, and always insisted on the rule of "ladies first", when entering a room, being served at meals or taking any privilege. The boy had no playmates, save one who was (in the eyes of mother and aunt) of inferior social standing. They deliberately kept Jack away from this boy, because of his "bad influence". Jack's name for his genital was "rudy", and for urination, "to be excused". From these facts, and other indications in my knowledge of the mother, it appeared that she had a certain amount of unconscious hostility towards sexuality, and in particular towards the boy's maleness.

The major fact of the boy's life was that he had no father of his own. Consciously, he spoke of having one father and two mothers, since he lived with his mother, aunt and uncle, and called this uncle "Daddy". He often heard his mother and aunt speak of his father's illness and death, and the difference this had made to his mother's life. When he went to the convent the year before, the nuns had spoken to him of his "other Daddy" who was "in Heaven". The boy had replied: "No, I have one Daddy and two Mummies"; but the nuns had insisted that he had "another Daddy in Heaven", where he was "very happy". Jack's mother told me this. Later on, I surmised from analytic material that the nuns had said that his father sang hymns in Heaven.

The aunt told me that Jack's mother was herself liable to fits of hysterical anger with the boy, the two shouting and storming at each other like two children. There was a certain amount of tension between the sisters about the boy (as I could see); but affection and helpfulness as well. The aunt envied the mother for her child; the mother envied the aunt for her husband and home and freedom from the necessity to go out to inferior work.

The boy slept in the same room as his uncle, the two women sharing another room. Jack often left his own bed in the night and insisted on getting into his uncle's.

Apart from the inhibiting effect of the mother's prudishness and her attitude towards his maleness, the central psychological problem of the boy's life was, in my judgement, that set up by his father's being dead and his uncle's having two women to look after.

MAIN OUTLINES OF THE ANALYSIS, PREVIOUS TO THE TRAUMATIC EVENTS

I do not propose to offer detailed material in this section, apart from one or two incidents; but chiefly to summarize the main themes.

(1) The boy was a naturally affectionate and confiding person, and began to show me his troubles as soon as he entered the room. From the toys on the table, he took up an engine and two coaches, and arranged these with one coach in front of and one behind the engine. He looked up at me enquiringly and, in a doubtful and rather sad tone, asked: "Engines *do* go like this, don't they? You *do* have a coach in front, don't you?" His tone showed that he did not quite believe it. I understood that he was, by his question, exploring my attitude towards him, as well as expressing some doubts about his mother and the situation at home.[1] In later hours, the action and query were repeated

---

[1] A technical question arises here: how far and in what way is it desirable, in analysing a young child, to make use in interpretations of knowledge about the patient's life and circumstances which has been gained from the parents or other adults?

In Jack's case, his mother actually said "Ladies first" to him in my presence and I saw his sheepish look at the time. But in my later interpretations I also referred to the fact of his father being dead, his living with aunt and uncle as well as mother, his mother having to go out to work, and other such circumstances—whenever I saw from the boy's play or conversation that these facts were indubitably at work in his mind, consciously or unconsciously.

At this age, and sometimes even at older ages, a child accepts it as quite natural and inevitable that his parents should have told the analyst such facts and events. He

several times, in different contexts, and with plenty of related material. I came presently to understand that his question had the following further meanings:—

(*a*) Jack was expressing his doubts, unhappiness and anxiety about the situation at home, where there were "one father and two mothers". (The coaches symbolically represented his mother and aunt; the engine, his father or uncle, as well as himself and the male genital.) He felt this "one father and two mothers" to be a bad arrangement, since the one man could not give both women all they needed, and the women quarrelled. Jack was puzzled, too, about the different circumstances of the two women. Why should one, his own "Mummy", have to go out to work to earn money and get tired and cross, whilst the other, his aunt "Mimi", could stay at home and have an easier time? Jack certainly connected the greater irritability and unhappiness of his mother with these harsh necessities. He felt that his uncle should give his mother, too, enough money to enable her to stay at home and be happy. The "one father and two mothers" meant not only that one father had to support and feed two mothers; unconsciously, it also meant that one man had to be potent enough for two mothers and satisfy them both genitally. He felt, too (as I realized later), that his own dead father, supposed to be happy singing hymns in heaven, ought to be in his home, working and helping his mother, bringing her money, saving her from work and unhappiness. The dead father, thus, was in the boy's mind selfish and cruel to his mother. This contributed to Jack's phantasies about his dead father, as a cruel and frightening figure.

(*b*) Jack was asking me whether "engines do *go* like this". It became clear that his mother's demand that "ladies should go first" was unconsciously associated in Jack's mind with her

---

will expect it to happen even more than it does. He does not resent it as an infringement of confidence or his rights as an individual, in the way an adolescent or an adult would do. Nevertheless, it stirs up persecutory fears of people leaguing together against him, and so on. These anxieties are relieved (*a*) by specific interpretation of them as such; (*b*) by the general relief which the child gains through the analytic use of the facts which the analyst knows, and the consequent understanding of what the child feels about these events; and (*c*) by the analyst's frank admission that the parents have told her these facts. Moreover, the child soon learns that the analyst does not tell the parents what happens in the analysis itself, nor make use, in a way hostile to the parents, of what the child shows her, the analyst. In other words, that the analyst does not in fact league either with the parents against the child or with the child against the parents. In these various ways, the child comes to feel that it is on the whole a helpful thing if the analyst has been told about external events and circumstances. Later on, he becomes able to communicate these external matters much more freely himself.

prudishness and her attitude towards sex. It was to him a depreciation of his manliness, an expression of her dislike and distrust of the penis, and of a wish to castrate him. In his query, he was wanting reassurance about this, and asking whether he could be potent in spite of "ladies going first".

(c) He was asking me whether I, too, had a hostile attitude to his maleness and thought women should have all the privileges; whether I, too, wanted to castrate him.

During the next few weeks, the further situations appearing in the analysis led to interpretations and conclusions as follows:—

(2) My interpretations about Jack's fear of being castrated by his mother and myself, and of the anxiety and hatred aroused in him by his mother's restrictive attitudes, and my references to his feelings about his uncle's difficulties with his mother and aunt, lessened the force of repression. This brought feelings of relief and a strong positive transference. As the boy's hate and suspicion became somewhat reduced, his positive feelings towards me developed, and his libidinal wishes towards his mother, and myself as representing her, began to appear. He could then bear to bring out more plainly the hatred itself, which he felt because of his direct sexual feelings being frustrated.

(3) Very soon, however, these Œdipus wishes brought up his fear of his uncle, and severe castration anxieties in reference to him. These anxieties drove him to feelings of submission to his uncle, and strengthened the masochistic feminine wishes of the inverted Œdipus situation. (Towards the end of the first week, Jack burnt his wrist on his uncle's cigarette, as he sat affectionately on his knee.) When these homosexual wishes were interpreted, together with their use as a defence against the dread arising from the heterosexual aims, his direct Œdipus wishes to his mother and myself came up again. The boy's libidinal aims moved to and fro between the heterosexual and homosexual positions, as interpretation relieved each set of anxieties as they came up in turn.

(4) Moreover, early oral wishes towards the penis, and the earliest homosexual aims, came into the open. The desire to incorporate the penis, orally and anally, with all its attendant phantasies of an internalized "good" and "bad" penis, was dramatized in Jack's analytic play. When he felt he had incorporated a good penis, he had hopes of being potent himself and achieving his heterosexual aims successfully. When he felt he had

internalized a destructive penis, he felt he became helpless and castrated. And these feelings of potency or of being castrated influenced his reparation phantasies. He felt that if he had a good internal penis, he could restore his mother and satisfy her sexually; conversely, when his internalized penis seemed bad, he despaired about making his mother well and happy.

The circumstances of his life emphasized Jack's emotional dependence upon his uncle, who was certainly a less restricting person than the two women—provided that the boy was "good", not over-assertive or demanding. The quarrels between mother and aunt also encouraged his homosexual attachment to his uncle. In his uncle, he sought a good father, so much needed to help him, both in his external life and in his internal problems. When he went into his uncle's bed at night, he was not only drawn by love and admiration, but also driven by the dread of the bad internalized penis, and of the quarrelling women. He had a great wish to feel that his uncle was a good friend; but the possibility of a desexualized friendly relationship was much hampered by his anxieties concerning the destructive internalized penis.

(5) The early loss of the boy's actual father, not seeing and knowing him as an external figure, had enhanced all his phantasies about the internalized father and given them particular features. The internal father was a dead and frightening figure,[1] In the course of the analysis, an intense longing to bring his father back to life, either in actuality or as an internal object, began to find expression.

(6) The boy's masturbation phantasies began to appear, with all their wishes, aggressions and anxieties. In one session, Jack brought a stuffed dog which he called "Pluto" (from the Mickey Mouse films) and made him "come alive" (as he said) by dancing and jigging him about on the couch—just as Jack himself jigged about in his moments of "queer" excitement. Jigging "Pluto" about represented masturbation, and showed the link between Jack's own jigging about in his "queer" excitement and his masturbation. When I interpreted the jigging as masturbation, Jack told me he played with his genital in the lavatory. But since

---

[1] Melanie Klein and Joan Riviere both tell me that they have seen how, in several cases, the death or disappearance of the father in the early years of the child has had a profound influence upon phantasies about the internalized father, as well as upon the development of the Œdipus complex. The internal father figure tends to be endowed with extreme qualities, the phantasy of an idealized internal father and that of an extremely sadistic one are both strengthened, and both in their turn reinforce the inverted Œdipus situation.

he spoke of "Pluto" "coming alive", the jigging about and the masturbation appeared to be also ways of reviving the internalized father and making him "come alive". It seemed that one of Jack's masturbation phantasies was this reviving of his dead (internalized) father in a good union with his mother.

(7) Jack's anxiety about being castrated by his mother and uncle because of his masturbation, his fear of his uncle's jealousy if his father did "come alive" inside him and he thus became potent, was also shown more definitely. He was afraid, too, of his mother's jealousy of me (of which there were signs in her manner to me, after the boy showed some improvement). These fears brought up hatred of both mother and uncle. His hate stirred aggressive impulses and the wish to attack mother and uncle with his erect "burning" penis and hot "burning" urine.[1] His earliest phantasies of the potent erect penis as a weapon of attack were revived, reawakening also his anxieties about the sadistic sexual intercourse of the internalized parents. When these latter phantasies were predominant, sexuality seemed bad in every respect.

(8) An important theme during the second to the fifth weeks was Jack's phantasies about his loud shouting voice. He had great pleasure in loud shouting, not gratified at home. Moreover, he felt that this voice, in screaming and shouting, could produce very unpleasant effects in the outer world—"horrible headaches", earaches, "black faces" and frowns in the people around him. His loud shouting at me made him fear my voice in turn—lest I should shout at him, even injure him and put "black" things into him, in revenge for his attack on me. My voice would accuse and reproach him and make him feel guilty. Here he projected on to me the voices of his internalized father, uncle and mother (super-ego).

One aspect of his feelings about his voice was his defiant use of forbidden "dirty" words, learnt from the forbidden playmate. These words also made people's faces "black", and were identified with his fæces and flatus and the destructive internal penis.

His pleasure and relief at being allowed to shout in the analysis alternated with doubts about my goodness and wisdom in letting him do these forbidden things, with his fear of seduction by me on account of this, and with dread of his own uncontrollable desires.

---

[1]Compare his remark, quoted on p. 20, about his own "bad gas" which had "all flared up and burnt" his father.

The analysis of these various psychological situations, and in particular of the masturbation phantasies, was proceeding in a normal way, when, in the sixth week of the analysis, a series of events occurred, extremely trying for the boy, and giving rise to acute anxieties.

TRAUMATIC EVENTS

These events were:—

(1) At the beginning of the week, Jack's aunt fell from a chair when reaching up to a high shelf and cut her wrist severely on a glass dish, severing an artery and tendons. The boy was in the room at the time, and saw and heard the crash. I surmised from associated material that he had been singing at the time of her fall. His mother told me in the boy's presence that his aunt had "nearly severed her wrist".

(2) This week was the anniversary of his father's death, which influenced his mother's state of mind (and probably his aunt's) and the talk which the boy heard, hence affecting his own trend of feeling and thinking.

(3) The third happening was that his grandmother, his mother's mother, was to be sent into hospital for an operation for cataract. This actually took place the following week, but was discussed in the boy's presence at home during this time. The grandmother was a very good friend to the boy and his mother. She helped them financially and thus often stood in the rôle of a father, in the boy's mind.

(4) The fourth event of the week, probably brought about by these other happenings, was that Jack's mother herself, when at work, dropped a large pot of boiling tea on her foot and scalded it severely.

Throughout these events, and during the next week or two, Jack missed many analytic sessions through his family circumstances.

THE ANALYSIS OF RESULTING ANXIETIES

The day after his aunt's accident Jack came into the analytic room as if he had not a care in the world, singing and playing rather defiantly and demonstratively; but after a few minutes he suddenly said "I *must not* sing", with much emphasis. This was followed by an outburst of aggression towards me, in which he re-enacted his aunt's accident and showed me that he felt he had caused her to fall and hurt herself. He threw a great deal of water about and flooded the floor, whilst standing on top of the chest of drawers. In this aggressive play, which represented the crash of his aunt's fall and the flowing blood, he gained much relief for the pent-up feelings which had no outlet at home, and much pleasure in aggressive conduct.

Presently, however, he showed me another aspect of his feelings in this hour. He reproached me openly for wearing (as I happened to be doing) a new frock on this day, the day after his aunt was injured; and threw wet dirty rags at my frock.

This wetting of my frock partly represented an aggressive attack with urine, but it seemed to be also a way of making me sorrow for his aunt's injury, as he could not bear to do himself. It showed me the stress which was caused in him by the demand of his mother and aunt that he should not shout or sing—"I *must not* sing". This prohibition stirred both anger and anxiety in him, since it made him feel more guilty about his aggressive tendencies and more deceitful if he had to hide them. Not only so: if he "must not sing", this took away his manic assertion of gaiety and cheerfulness and denial of sorrow and depression, and delivered him up to the latter feelings which he could not bear. So the flowing water and the wet put upon me also represented the tears which he felt *he* was expected to shed for his aunt's hurts. I was to sorrow instead of him. But then, after he had wet me, not being able to bear to see his own grief represented through me and the suffering he had put upon me, he hated me for that, too, and attacked me because of it.

Thus Jack began the hour by denying any distress or anxiety or any occasion for such feelings. His defiant manner showed that he expected me to reproach him or revenge his aunt's hurt. As I did not do so, he could express his sense of guilt in the voice of mother or aunt (internalized): "I *must not* sing". Then he could show me how aggressive he had felt and what harm he had done, re-enacting the scene. This in its turn brought up anxiety and guilt towards me about being so aggressive in my room—flooding it, etc. He dealt with this first by projecting guilt and callousness on to me—I ought not to wear a new frock. I should suffer with or instead of him. But then he had to attack me as a suffering person. The suffering loved object (primarily internal) which cannot be made happy and well must be attacked and killed, so that the ego may be spared the intolerable pain and conflict of the experience. (There is a close connection here with suicide impulses, as will be seen later.)

Jack's anxiety on leaving me that day was considerable, both because of the frightening situation at home, and because he feared that, in his aggression towards me and his wish to make me suffer, he had actually damaged me, too.

The following morning he had violent tantrums at home, and did not want to come to see me. However, he did come; and in this and the following hour the conflict between his destructive wishes and his desire to save people—e.g. from drowning and burning—was worked out dramatically.

For instance, he made a ship with chairs, and I was to sit in it and be kept "safe" from floods and storms. The ship represented an omnipotent means of controlling his storms of hatred and disastrous floods of urine. Later, he showed that he wanted me to help him preserve his mother from harm, by helping him to be clean and control his urine and fæces. He put a towel on the chair where he was to sit, calling it a "nappy". Later still, he pretended that all the toys and small objects in his drawer were "coal", and said he would "cart all the coal away" and "make it all tidy" (i.e. all the dead, dirty black things, the destructive fæces).

His early anxieties about destructive wetting and dirtying had thus come up again in response to the happenings at home. He felt such aggression in himself to be responsible for all the bad happenings in his world. (As Melanie Klein's work has shown, the child uses his anal and urethral bodily functions as an instrument of his sadistic impulses towards his mother, and feels them to be all-powerful in destruction.)

He had brought "Pluto" with him again, also a boat and a "Mickey Mouse" (these standing for father, mother and son); and he showed me in various ways his wish to make his aunt better and to give her many children. At the end of the hour he tried in a friendly but omnipotent way to save me from the danger of his destructive tendencies by getting me to go first out of the room ("ladies first"), leaving him standing on top of the chest of drawers shouting very loudly. In this way, he proved that, although he made a loud noise as he had been doing when his aunt fell, I would nevertheless be able to walk out uninjured. When he came out of the play-room, he told his mother that "Pluto", who had been sitting on the couch all the hour, had "been weeping his eyes out"; and he added, about "Pluto's" supposed weeping, "That's sorry for Granny". "Pluto", in this case, stood for one aspect of himself—when he was feeling the grief and guilt which he had tried to defend himself against in various ways.

In his play during these two hours, he had swung between the following situations: (*a*) saving me (his mother) from urinary attacks by making a ship; (*b*) attempts to undo past aggression by preventing himself, and making me prevent him, from dirtying the chair, etc.; (*c*) projecting out of his inner world the dangerous fæces and bits of people represented by "coal"—everything had become black coal and must be carted away and tidied up; (*d*) reviving his father and bringing about a happy family situation, in which he and his father, together or alternately ("Pluto" and "Mickey" and the boat) gave his mother children. This not only satisfied his libidinal wishes but also made use of his potency in acts of reparation; (*e*) magically and omnipotently controlling me and my actions, as standing for the injured aunt and mother— this was particularly at the end of the hour; (*f*) making "Pluto" "weep his eyes out", as representing himself when he was grieving. In all these ways he was trying to keep his guilt and depression at bay and overcome them, and at times was expressing his wishes. In his remarks to his mother when he left, Jack's sorrow and depression were fully shown—one aspect of these being his feeling that the only way to make his grandmother's eyes better was to weep his own eyes out. The comment to his mother was also an attempt, partly conscious, partly unconscious, to show her that he *was* sorry for his grandmother, and thus reconcile himself to her; but it also expressed the actual grief and guilt which he had tried to overcome during the hour. The analytic work of these hours had rendered him more capable of bearing and of expressing his grief.

That same evening, Jack's mother scalded herself, and he was not able to return to me for a week, since his aunt was now busy caring for his mother. When he came back, he at once reproached me grievously for not "keeping things right". He ran his toy engine along a straight join in the top of the table, saying most reproachfully to me: "Why didn't you know that engines should run on rails? Why didn't you keep it straight?" Here he defended himself against his own guilt and grief about his mother's accident by projecting responsibility on to me. He showed me again in a number of ways what distress he felt at this further accident, in what despair he was at not being able to prevent these awful happenings and how terrified he was of his own aggression. He felt he should have kept his mother (and his aunt and grandmother) safe; unconsciously, this extended to phantasies about his parents' sexual intercourse.

When I spoke of these phantasies, he began to sing a song, one which appeared a good deal during the next few weeks, about a "lover" who "yesterday went away". He sang, "They asked me how I knew my own true love was true"—a song which ends "smoke gets in your eyes". To his mind, the "smoke" meant both the "black stuff" (fæces), used as an instrument of hate, which had hurt his grandmother's eyes, and the tears which he ought to shed to make them better, but which would thus darken his own vision. But to cry meant nothing short of "crying his eyes out" (as he had said about "Pluto" the day before); and this meant both being blinded and castrated. His castration anxieties were linked with his depression. But the song about the "lover who yesterday went away" expressed his longing for the return of his father, and the feeling that it was the loss of his actual father (and a good internal father) which had led to these disasters, to the distresses of mother and aunt and grandmother. He could show me his sadness at the loss of the helping father and his longing for his return, after his anxiety was relieved by my interpreting to him how he was projecting his guilt and responsibility on to me.

The next week, the seventh of the analysis, brought the following major responses. At the beginning of the week, his grandmother went into hospital and was successfully operated upon. The day she went, he was very sad and depressed, and showed his castration anxieties in many details of his play. When I said he was sad because so many hurtful things had happened which he felt he could not prevent or make better, he told me: "Grannie gone away". He then got on to the couch, right under the fitted cover, and shouted at me from under it. Later on, he asked me to lie under the cover in the same way, when he tried to jump on me and to kick and trample my face. (I did not, of course, allow him to carry this to the point of hurting me.) He was now representing his blinded grandmother (being under the cover), and the operation on her eyes, which he felt to be a cruel assault (the kicking and trampling).

Thus, he first showed me how he identified himself with his blinded grandmother (in unconscious phantasy, he contained her); and then represented himself as carrying out the operation upon me (as standing for her). The operation itself represented a sadistic primal scene. (As will appear, next day he asked me to "wake him up" by running a toy engine and trucks over him when he was under the cover—a reference to being wakened up by intercourse between uncle and aunt when at one time he had slept in their room.) He wanted to be the surgeon who would restore her sight by the operation; but the severity of the boy's conflicts is shown in his acting out the operation as a cruel kicking and trampling. And just as he felt the operation, intended to restore and heal, to be yet cruelly damaging and painful, so, in his phantasies, sexual intercourse, giving life and pleasure, was yet a cruel and dangerous happening, which might lead to castration and even death.

These interpretations lessened his anxiety somewhat, and as a result his aggression and sadism were modified to some degree. He now acted out his grandmother's experiences by playing at being a barking, biting dog, pretending to bite me, and saying: "I'm a little dog". The biting dog stood for the surgeon's knife, as well as for his own teeth and oral aggression, the barking for his loud aggressive shouting, with which he had often annoyed and hurt his mother and grandmother. (As I mentioned earlier, his own aggressive voice was equated with a destructive internal penis and bad father.) He thus acted out both his own aggression and that of the sadistic father—now represented by the surgeon operating on his grandmother.

The next day, after much further play of biting me like a dog, and some attempts to do so actually, Jack hid under the cover of the couch again, and got me to "wake him up" by running a toy engine and trucks over him. He then said, "I'm ill in bed"; but he could not bear to act this out, and had at once to get up and laugh and shout. Instead, then, I had to "be Granny", ill in bed. He now put many little toys, engines, etc., near to me for me to look at, to comfort me and prove that I was not blind. When I lay still, representing the ill grandmother, he became very quiet and subdued. Then, suddenly, with obvious relief, he said: "I found out it was only Mrs. Isaacs"—thus comforting himself with the reality that we were only pretending, and that I was not in fact ill or blind. Thus the immediate effect of the interpretations was to lessen the phantastic elements in the situation and foster the more realistic aspect. This is an example of the way in which a purely analytic procedure of interpreting unconscious phantasies and anxieties promotes the sense of reality.

Jack then threw and poured water on to the floor, became a "big Daddy showing the babies how to skate" (pretended babies) on the floor. He struggled hard to control the amount of water which ran off the table on to the floor, holding a vessel underneath to catch the drips, and saying: "I'm being a sailor saving the babies". Then he gave many gifts to "one of the babies" (now a small doll), as he had done to me when I represented the ill grandmother. The ill grandmother (thought by him to be dying) had thus now changed into a growing baby—a more hopeful figure. (The well-known "reversal of generations" phantasy.)

He now put little toy people into the largest basin of water, calling them "the babies". He put them close together and said: "Now they're cuddling each other". The babies now represented the parents re-created and loving, in a good sexual intercourse. The basin represented his body, and the babies (parents) were also internal. He made a nail-brush into a "raft" for the babies to float upon, with many other details which showed his wish to save his grandmother, re-creating her as well as his parents, in the babies, by means of his good creative penis, the "raft".

In these two hours, thus, we see, first, a short-lived defence against depression (his accusations against me, followed by his biting attacks, acting out the aggressive impulses); then, an open depression, with the feeling that *he* had now to suffer what his grandmother was suffering. He had internalized his grandmother, as a blinded and tortured and thus also a persecuting object; (and she, as we already know, also stood for the mother, castrated and injured in a dangerous sexual intercourse with father.) Then he projected this internal suffering grandmother on to me, and I had to go through her suffering, whilst he was the powerful sadistic father, biting, cutting, burning, blinding me and rendering me helpless. (At this stage, he had little hope that the operation on grandmother's eyes would actually heal and restore her sight.) Then, once again, the depression arising from his concern about the suffering of his grandmother, and from the internalization of the injured grandmother, returned; this was once more dealt with by projecting her on to me and making me play her part instead.

This was also a way of controlling me (and her), as an external object. The injured object is necessarily dangerous and must be controlled. He showed this intense need to control by his watching and ordering every detail of my actions, and his feverish efforts at this point to control the water running down from the table, etc. The very intensity of his efforts showed how strong were his recurrent doubts about the possibility of controlling his own and his internal father's aggression. But presently, as a result of the interpretation of his aggressive wishes and his anxieties about them, his hate and sadism were reduced, and trust and confidence in himself grew somewhat stronger. This meant that he, as well as his father, could have a good union with his mother, and that his penis could be life-giving and life-saving. (He had said: "I'm being a sailor saving the babies.")   He began to feel, through the analysis, that he was incorporating, and had in the past incorporated, a good penis, a good father, potent to heal and save. He could comfort the ill grandmother with his gifts, could save the babies and re-create the internalized grandmother in the babies. The release of his libido, along with the lessening of anxiety about the internalized parents, brought with it also an improvement in his sense of reality— as was shown in his comment: "I found out it was only Mrs. Isaacs".

During the next day or two, Jack was told that his grandmother's operation had been successful. This was a great reassurance to him. It meant to him that she would not die, but would be able to see again and would come back to him as a good friend. Together with my interpretations, it enabled him now to bring out more fully and vividly in the analysis his feelings of guilt and responsibility towards his grandmother, as well as his anxieties about his dead father and his own inside. Owing to the lessening of anxiety through the analytic work, his phantasies could now become manifest, and be worked over and tested in reality. But their content as it appeared in the material of the hours which followed showed what a formidable experience the boy was undertaking.

In the middle of the week, Jack made many attempts to wash the floor and the wall, which he called "Granny's bottom", actually chanting these words as he did it. But his attempts to clean things and make them look better resulted in an ever greater mess, and suddenly he urinated on the floor. This change of attitude, as could be seen in the expression of his face, came about when he realized that his constructive efforts were proving vain. It was his despair at making a mess with the soap and water when he was trying to clean the wall (which stood for his mother's and the analyst's, as well as his grandmother's, bottom) which led to the actual urination. This lack of skill denoted to Jack that he could not use his fæces and urine as gifts, as a means of cleaning and restoring his loved persons; their destructive qualities seemed to be too powerful. There was then nothing left but to regress to the anal level of defiant dirtying, and a distrust of his helpful wishes. This is a common situation with little children in ordinary life, too. With Jack, whose anxieties about dangerous excrements were so pronounced, and were fostered by his strict environment, it was indeed a major disaster to find that he could not make a constructive use of his fæces and urine, represented by soap and water.

Presently, when scrubbing the floor, he said, "I'm washing Daddy's tummy"; and in the middle of the soapy mess, he drew a face with the lather, calling it "Daddy's face". (Father's face in the middle of father's "tummy" represented father inside his own body.) He told me: "He's smiling"; but his tone and manner showed his scepticism about his smiling—about his father's being "happy in Heaven", as the nuns had said—as well as his doubts about the internalized father. Since he cannot keep his father happy inside himself, safe from his own fæces and aggression, he cannot believe that he could be happy in Heaven. (In the unconscious mind, Heaven, the place furthest away, means the place nearest but least able to be explored, viz.: one's own inside.)

The next day, he told me that it was his own "bad gas", the "bad gas in me", which had hurt his Daddy and killed him. It had, he said, "all flared up and burnt him". (This was an entirely spontaneous reference to flatus; I had not mentioned it in my interpretations.) Here we have a clear expression of Jack's fear that the good objects inside him, the helpful father, had been or would be destroyed by his fæces and flatus. (It was partly because of this danger that his internalized grandmother had had to be projected on to me, in the play of the previous days; to keep her safe from his excrements.)

After this he tried to "make me better" (as representing his mother and grandmother) by giving me "tea" to drink (actually water). But this was quickly followed by dropping the cup and flooding the floor with water, and then by actual urination. Since his excrements were felt to be so dangerous—so much so that they had "burnt up" his father inside him—they could not be relied upon to satisfy and restore me (his mother and grandmother). This despair led once again to a regressive wetting. (Such fears are commonly operative in the familiar difficulties shown by many children in accepting habit-training, or in causing a later regression to wetting and dirtying after clean habits have been established.)

In these two hours, we see the open expression of Jack's phantasies about the destructive qualities of his urine and fæces and flatus, with admission of guilt and responsibility, associated with the attempts to restore his injured grandmother and mother (myself) by washing and feeding us, and to bring his father to life again (making him smile in his drawing)—alternating with hopelessness and a regressive sadism, when his lack of skill, the weakness of his ego, brought up overwhelmingly his doubts about the possibility of such reparation.

Once again, now, Jack's Œdipus wishes came forward, together with his phantasies about his mother and myself as external objects. He was now more able to show me something of his interest in her genital, and his anxieties about it. Sitting on the floor beside me, he asked me to show him my "leg and knees", saying pleadingly: "There's a good girl". When I refused to do this, he put a series of toy cars and coal trucks in one long line, saying "It's your rudy". Thus he tried to prove that I had a penis, was not castrated as he feared. In other ways he showed me that he feared not only that my genital (representing his mother's) was injured and lacked a penis, but also that it was full of "dirty black stuff" (fæces) and a dangerous father's penis. His early phantasies, derived from his own aggressive wishes towards his mother's body, were now stirred again. His sexual wish to see his mother's genital, and to have intercourse with her, was much reinforced by these anxieties and his need to get reassurance about them. It was this need which made his pleading so urgent and the frustration of his libidinal desire to see my genital so severe.

During the next few days, Jack had to stay away from the

analysis, because of his mother's having to go out to do extra
work, in order to earn more money for herself and the boy. When
he returned, he spoke to me of the bandages on his grandmother's
eyes, he having been to see her in hospital. To him, it seemed
that her head was hurt as well, since the bandages went round her
head. He spoke of it in a context which, following on the previous
hour when he had so much wanted to see my genital and prove
it was not injured, led me to infer that he had also seen his
mother's sanitary towels at some time. To Jack's mind these were
bandages on an injury, too, and confirmed his fears that her
body and her genital were hurt and damaged.

He now burnt a lot of paper in the hearth, and then stamped
on the burnt paper, saying "It's dead now". Then he hit his own
head with a railway coach, and fell down on the floor, saying
"Now *I'm* dead". (This linked with the bandages round his
grandmother's head.)

The sight of his grandmother's bandaged head had aroused his
castration fears in an extreme degree. The threat of castration
struck him as something which really happens. (*Cf.* the myth
of the head of Medusa, and Freud's view as to the traumatic
effect of the sight of the female genital.) His phantasies about the
destructive nature of sexual intercourse seemed to him to be
confirmed. The father (the surgeon) castrated the mother
(grandmother's bandaged head, mother's menstruation). Moreover, the injured female genital was a direct threat to his own
penis, as he showed by hitting his own head with the railway
coach, which in his play had stood for his mother. But he was
inextricably involved in the parents' sadistic intercourse; his
head represented his own penis, the father's penis and the mother's
genital (grandmother's bandaged head). I interpreted his
castration fears, and the complex situation of mutual castration
by the sadistic parents felt to be inside himself, with the resulting
threat to his own body. He responded to these interpretations,
then, by playing at being a "kind lion". "Now I'm a kind lion",
he said. That is to say, he had to some extent overcome the danger
of castration; his own penis, and that of his internal father, were
now felt to be potent but friendly. That some doubt still remained,
however, was shown by what followed. At the end of the hour,
he took home some toy soldiers from the play-room, and in the
waiting room he showed these to his mother, asking her: "*Why*
does Mrs. Isaacs let me take soldiers home?"

In this hour, we see how his anxieties had become more acute again, by reason of (a) his seeing his grandmother bandaged in hospital, (b) the fact that, because of the cost of her operation, his mother had to work still harder and (c) his enforced absence from the analysis. My interpretations somewhat relieved his anxieties, so that he could feel that his genital was less threatened, and that the internalized father became less sadistic and dangerous, a "kind lion". This "kind lion" was a modification (through the release of libido) of the cruel internal father. Jack's question to his mother at the end of the hour, however (which I interpreted to him the following day) showed that his doubts were still active. He was warning his mother that I, the analyst, was being too lenient with him (as he feared), seducing him and allowing his dangerous wishes to come into the open. I myself was also the kind but suspect lion-father (who was still a "lion", although a kind one); and Jack was warning his mother that this supposedly kind father was still a danger to her. And I, the lion-father, was being blamed for Jack's own aggression.

The sight of his grandmother bandaged in hospital had been the climax to the series of frightening and distressing events during the previous fortnight, in which mother, aunt and grandmother had all suffered serious hurt. These happenings had stirred up in him intense anxieties of a psychotic nature, referring to the primal scene between the internalized parents. The "burning" and biting father's penis ("Pluto" having changed into a "lion"), and the boy's own "burning" urine and destructive faeces were felt to constitute a threat not only to the internalized mother but also to his own eyes, head and genital. The struggle with the lion-father, the attempt to kill him, itself brought death to his own body. These are some of the psychotic anxieties which Melanie Klein (1932 and 1935) has described as operating in the early mental life of the child. Normally, they become worked over and greatly modified in the course of development, but if they are (owing to various influences) retained in full strength, they form the potential nucleus of an open psychosis in later life.

Jack brought some of the soldiers back next day in a paper bag. He took the soldiers out and burnt the bag, then stamped the flames out, saying "Now it's dead", and, "Aren't we having a *lovely* bonfire?" Later, he threatened to burn me with the burning paper. The bag stood for his own body and penis, containing the

dangerous burning penis of the father, and he was showing me his
sadistic desires and pleasure in destroying the father and his
penis with his burning urine.   His manner showed, however,
that his pleasure in destruction was being over-emphasized, to
cover up his great anxiety about experiencing in his own body
the fight between the burning penis of father and his own burning
urine.

In terms of the primary instincts, he was showing in these
actions and threats his need to deflect outward the destructive
impulses (the death instinct); in terms of emotional experience,
he was urgently trying to get these frightening objects and events
outside himself, because of his overwhelming anxiety about
internal dangers.   He felt, when in the grip of these phantasies,
that all he could do with external objects was to destroy them—
the bag, the flames, myself.

When I interpreted to him his anxieties about the burning
internal penis and his reasons for wishing to attack me with it,
he suddenly and quickly took off all his garments, except his
shoes and socks, and stood naked with an erect penis.   Finally, he
took off his socks and shoes, too, saying "In case my feet are black".
(Probably the intention to unclothe and exhibit himself had
already been in his mind, unconsciously, when the previous day
he had asked his mother "why I let him" take the soldiers home.)
In saying "In case my feet are black", Jack was justifying his
nakedness in my (and his mother's) eyes, and displacing his
anxiety and our possible disapproval from his genital to his feet.
But he was also showing that there was a further meaning, hinted
at now in his tones and gestures, but coming out more clearly in
later material: viz. that nothing must be left covered up, hidden
or secret, in case it was dirty or bad, and we were thus deceived
and in danger.   It was partly his anxiety about the dirty and
dangerous character of his genital—it might burn or flood me
with destructive urine—which made him feel so imperative a
need to show it to me.   I interpreted these feelings to him, whilst
he ran about the room triumphantly for a time.

When, presently, I asked him to dress again, he became very
angry with me. He said emphatically "But I *like* being undressed",
and rushed about the room shouting.   When I persisted, he
became anxious and most obstinately refused.   When I held out
his garments to him, he rushed away from me as if I were going
to punish or hurt him.   When, after some further interpretation

of his fears, I again urged him to dress, his anxiety became over-whelming. He went and lay down on top of the chest of drawers, covering himself all over with the cloths which he had (on previous days) used for wiping the floor and washing the wall ("Daddy's tummy" and "Granny's bottom").   When he covered himself with these cloths, therefore, he represented the injured grand-mother and dead father. He lay very still, as if lifeless. When, for practical reasons, I once more asked him to put his clothes on, he became extremely angry, and tried to bite me in his rage. Then he said: "There's lions and tigers and walruses in the room", looking about him in a way which showed that to him the room actually was full of these threatening animals. I told him that these fierce animals represented me; in his mind, I was now certain to bite him in revenge, because he had tried to do this to me in his anger with me. This interpretation relieved him enough for him to be able to obey my request, and (with my help) get dressed and leave in a fairly calm state of mind.

The following session, he wanted to undress as soon as he arrived; I refused to agree (partly because it was cold weather and he had so recently had an attack of pneumonia); whereupon he became defiant. He then burnt a lot of paper in the hearth, urinated on the floor and mixed up the burnt paper with the urine (and water) on the floor, making a black mess all over the floor. Having failed to change my mind by his defiance, he now tried other means. He went to the lavatory and defæcated, coming back to me and saying in a confident and coaxing tone: "*Now* I will undress!" Evidently he felt quite certain that now he had got rid of the dangerous objects from his inside, I should let him undress. When I again said "No", he once more said there were "lions in the room", looking at these "lions" and hitting out at them, with such a fixed and intense gaze as to make it quite certain that he had a definite hallucination, seeing them clearly and objectively. My unwillingness to let him undress had been taken by him to mean that he had *not* been able to leave the "lions" (destructive fæces and dangerous internalized penis) safely in the lavatory, as well as that I would not let him have the pleasure and reassurance he was seeking; and this made him want to bite me like a lion, and then again fear my revenge. I told him that these fierce "lions" not only stood for me and the vengeful attack he feared I should make upon him, but also for the lion-father (no longer "kind") inside himself. He felt he *must* get this threatening father's penis outside himself, since his own body was in such danger from it. If I let him run about naked and show me his genital, and thus prove (as he felt) that his nakedness did not harm me, that I was not burnt up by exposure to his penis, this reassured him about what was going on in secret inside him. But when I refused to let him undress, he felt that I was actually prohibiting nakedness as such. This seemed to confirm his fears about having a dangerous father's penis inside him and could not be endured. He therefore defended himself against this overwhelming dread by projecting the dangerous father outside as the hallucinated lions and tigers.

In these two hours, we see Jack's psychotic anxieties about the destructive contents of his body, and what was going on inside it, come to open expression. He attempted to deal with these dangerous objects and events in various ways: (a) by projecting them out of his body and annihilating them (symbolically, by taking the soldiers out of the bag, burning the bag and "killing" the flames; literally, by defæcating and urinating); (b) by manically *denying* danger and badness in his triumphant nakedness, and putting this denial to the test.

His obsessional need to unclothe his body and exhibit his genital arose from complex sources: the fear of the external castrating father (his uncle) and mother, who must be defied; the anxiety and distress that his genital was dirty, disgusting and dangerous to his mother (myself); the dread of the bad internalized penis and his own fæces and urine. These will act through the boy's external genital to damage the mother's body. His genital must therefore not be left hidden, but must be brought into the open, to be controlled by his own eyes and those of the analyst. In addition, the act of taking off the clothes had itself a meaning in relation to Jack's anxieties about the inside of his body. Melanie Klein has found (and my own experience confirms) that clothes, which come close round the body, affect its comfort so much and are soiled by it, can often represent the contents of the body itself. The act of undressing thus meant not only uncovering the outside of the body to prove that it was clean and not harmful, but also getting rid of the disgusting and evil things inside it.[1]

When I did not allow Jack to gain in this particular way the reassurance he sought against his overwhelming anxieties, he

---

[1] These motives enter into the drive to exhibitionism, generally. I have found them at work with adult patients.

showed me what would happen to him if he were left at the mercy
of the dangerous internalized parents and the bad substances
inside him; he, too, would lie dying like his grandmother (he still
feared she would die) covered up with bandages, dirty cloths and
fæces; or dead like his father in the grave. And when, on the
earlier occasion on which he had undressed, I urged him to get
up and dress, he showed me that, in order to be able to come to
life, he would have to turn his aggression outwards and, in the
rôle of the lion-father towards me, would bite me in his rage.
This was followed instantly by his fear of my biting him in revenge,
and then by the hallucination of the "lions and tigers and walruses", representing both myself and the dangerous internalized
father, now perceived in the outside world. (I shall discuss the
meaning of the hallucination more fully at a later point.)

The following day Jack again begged me to let him undress.
When I refused, he scrubbed the floor and drank some of the
dirty water. Then he sang the song "Baa, Baa, black sheep",
shouting it very loudly and forcefully in a defiant manner. Here
he was taking in the dirty water (i.e. urine and fæces) in order to
show me how he had got dirty inside (he was the "black sheep")
and to reproach me for not letting him undress. He felt it was
my fault if he were so evil inside. In unconscious logic, my not
letting him get the bad things out was equivalent to my putting
them into him. The scrubbing of the floor was a sort of pleading
(like the "baa, baa" of the lamb): "See how much I want to
make my inside, and Granny's bottom, clean"—just as the
actual defæcation the day before had in part been a pleading and
a demonstration of the wish to be clean. All the more, therefore,
it was my fault if he were not. In terms of the life and death
instincts, the drinking of dirty water was an expression of the
despair which he felt when the good he so much desired (i.e.
nakedness approved of by me) seemed unattainable. If I withheld
the good things (life) from him, then he yielded to the bad, to
dirt (and death). The death instinct predominated.

In his song he now emphasized very much the words: "None
for the little boy who *used* to live down the lane". (That is, "no
wool" for him.) Now the boy playmate whom he was not allowed
to see, because he was "rude" and "dirty", a "black sheep",
had actually lived "down the lane" from Jack's home. Jack was
therefore showing me, not only his longing for his playmate, but
also his guilt towards him. The two had been parted because

they had done "rude" and "dirty" things together—played with dirt and exhibited to each other. Jack's guilt was made stronger by his being deprived of his ally. He felt the playmate had been sent away because they had made each other dirty. Hence he himself became all the more a "black sheep". His present urgent wish to exhibit his genital was partly a confession of the past behaviour which his mother and aunt considered so unforgivable. And his pleading with me in scrubbing the floor and singing, was asking me to help him bring his playmate back, and make him clean again.

But there was another detail of circumstance, which I may not quote, which showed indubitably that the boy who "*used* to live down the lane" and could not have any wool was also his own dead father. He, too, as well as the playmate, was "the lover who yesterday went away", in another song which Jack sang to me, as we saw earlier. It will be remembered that Jack had already told me that it was his own "bad gas" inside himself which had "all flared up and burnt" his father and killed him. He felt guilt towards his father, as well as towards his lost playmate. Jack wanted to revive and bring the father back, too, as he had already shown me in many ways. His urge to take off his clothes and exhibit his erect genital now, in so far as it meant getting the wicked and hurtful things out of his body, and undoing the harm done in the past, meant also restoring and winning back the "kind lion", the good father, external and internal.

The next day Jack again demanded that he should be allowed to undress, as soon as he came. I had now come to the conclusion that, in this particular case, I could not go on refusing his demand without disturbing his analysis seriously, or even stultifying it altogether. Here, again, we come to an important question of technique. Generally speaking, children, even at so young an age, express their wishes and anxieties in words or symbolically by play and gestures, and relief is obtained partly by acting out in play, partly through the moment-by-moment interpretations. Direct gratifications (e.g. exhibiting, masturbating, obtaining food, defæcating on the floor, and so on) are discouraged by the analyst. In Jack, the obsessional drive to undress himself in order to gain reassurance and to act out his aggressive and libidinal wishes was extremely strong—as all the material so far has shown. But the chief reasons why he could not obtain relief through a symbolic expression of his wish only were (*a*) the overwhelming anxieties caused by the traumatic events already described, so many in so short a space of time; and (*b*) the frequent absences from the analysis brought about by these events. These absences were, on the one hand, a great frustration; and on the other, they prevented the anxieties aroused by the traumatic events being dealt with step by step as they arose, and caused them to be heaped up until they became unbearable.

I therefore decided that it was wiser now to be quite neutral in this matter, and confine my comments to interpreting his compulsion to undress, and all the details of his actions. When I did not again say he must not, he at once took all his clothes off. He climbed up on the table, and defæcated there. The expression of his face was friendly and his tone of voice gentle, as he now said to me "Now wipe it up". I did this; and when the table was clean again, Jack took a black crayon and wrote letters and drew on the table—*the first time* he had written or drawn with any of the crayons during the analysis, so far. He evidently felt that if he were allowed to make a gift of his fæces to me, and I was willing to clear them away, he could feel a greater trust in himself and in me. This, together with my interpretations of his anal wishes and anxieties, was felt as a proof that the contents of his body were not so disgusting and dangerous to me, or to himself, as he had feared they would be. This also brought reassurance about the destructive character of the internalized father. Black marks made by him (and father) on the table (mother's body) could now be felt as good and useful things; he could sublimate his anal wishes in the effort to learn to write and draw.

In the next hour, Jack again undressed and then burnt a lot of paper, stamping the flames out "to kill them" and "to save you from being burnt", as he said. Then he sang a song about "something inside, which will not be denied, which I cannot hide". He put water on the floor and scrubbed the floor again with a soapy lather, calling himself a "gutter urchin". He played at shooting, begged me to "shoot him dead"; then crawled right under the hearth rug, asking me to walk on him as he lay there. (Needless to say, I did not do this.) After this, he again climbed on top of the chest of drawers, and lay there absolutely still, limp and seemingly lifeless, but with an erect penis, and naked save for the floor cloths which he again arranged over himself. When the time came to leave, he refused to have his legs washed clean—he had blackened them with the wet black paper.

In this hour, we see how he felt he had to attack and kill the burning internalized father's penis, to save me from being burnt by it. It was this which was hidden inside him, which "could not be denied". His request that I should "shoot him dead" and walk upon him, his calling himself a "gutter urchin", referred not only to himself, but also and mainly to the internalized father's penis, the "lions and tigers and walruses" which were such a threat to me and to himself. This penis must be killed, burnt up, shot and got rid of, to save me and himself from death. His suicidal aim (to be shot dead and trodden into the gutter) represented this attack upon the lion-father and burning father's penis inside him. In lying "dead" on the chest of drawers, he acted out the death of the internalized parents and his own death.

Freud (1917) has shown us how the self-abasement, the "shameless" protestations of worthlessness and longing to be punished of the melancholic, all his "delusional belittling" of himself, refer not only to the ego, but also to the introjected object: ". . . the self-reproaches are reproaches against a loved object which have been shifted on to the patient's own ego". This was patent in Jack's abasement and self-blame, and wish for punishment. Unconsciously, he blamed his father for his own destructiveness. In obstinately refusing to have his legs washed clean before going home, he showed that he felt this need for blame and punishment (unconsciously also his blame and reproaches against his internalized dead father) in relation to his actual mother as well as to me; he wanted her to appreciate what he had inside him, and so be warned of her own danger. It was also an expression of his guilt towards me, because he made such a mess in my room, and I had to work so hard to clean it up again.

The next day, he took off his clothes on arrival, urinated on the floor and pretended to "swim" in the urine. Then he burnt more paper, whilst singing the song about "smoke gets in your eyes". He made a great heap of the burnt paper, insisting that "it must *all* be burnt up" and got rid of. Then he blacked himself from top to toe with the burnt paper, and fished more black (soot, etc.) down the chimney with a broom. He said he was trying to "clean the chimney" (i.e. his own anus and mine, mother's and grandmother's); but in doing this, he got himself more black than ever. His impulse to clean himself and his objects was ambivalent.

In this hour, we see a regression to anal libido, occurring partly because the boy had had so little chance of satisfying these

impulses at the normal time in his ordinary life. But his insistence
that the paper "must *all* be burnt up" and got rid of, and other
signs of *anxiety*, showed that these activities were by no means
only a matter of libidinal gratification, but were also concerned
with getting rid of dangerous inner objects.

The following hour he again undressed, burnt paper and
blacked himself all over; then he asked for the broom again, with
which to "sweep down the chimney". I interpreted his wish to
incorporate (anally) a good penis (the broom to clean the
chimney), in order to counteract the evil one, already ruined
and made dangerous by his own "bad gas" and fæces, and to rid
his body of its destructive contents. I linked this wish to incorporate a good penis with the homosexual wishes (shown
earlier in the analysis) towards his uncle (as the live father); if the
uncle was a good father and friend to him, this also meant that he
had a good father inside him.

Later that day, his mother told me a detail which indirectly
confirmed this. He had been called a "gutter urchin" at home
one day, after he had muddied himself with the soil in his uncle's
garden. I have no doubt that his doing this, like his blacking
himself in the analysis, was a defiant and despairing messing of
himself, following on the fairlue of an attempt to do creative and
reparative work in the garden, as his uncle was doing. If he finds
he cannot garden skilfully and fruitfully, then in despair he
messes himself all over, to represent the evil inside, attack and
punish the internalized dead father.

A further detail which his mother told me linked with his
compulsion to undress. Jack had recently seen a cinema film
of little black boys in a sunny climate, naked and swimming and
singing merrily. He had been told that sun-bathing would make
one strong and well. Moreover, the song he often sang about
"they asked me how I knew my own true love was true" was
sung by a negro in a gramophone record of which mother and
aunt were fond. Jack had thus made use of these reassuring
notions—that to be naked and black meant being strong and
well and merry, and that mother and aunt liked what "black
men" sang—in an attempt to overcome his dread of the black
and dangerous substances, the "black man" (dead father) inside
him. But unconsciously he had not believed these things. They
served only as a means of *denying* his anxieties and unconscious
convictions, not of allaying them. And in his unremitting

insistence on being naked in the analysis, and going home with blackened legs, he had mocked at those who pretended that naked black boys are happy and well. He felt it to be only a pretence, just as he felt it to be a pretence and a lie that his dead father was happy and sang hymns in Heaven. He felt they ought *not* to be happy and well, if they were black. For him, the "black man" inside was a dangerous monster, a lion or a tiger.

The analysis, during the last few days, of Jack's compulsion to undress, and of the reparative element in his homosexual wishes towards his uncle, enabled him to do without actually undressing after this day.

The following week, Jack had again to stay away from the analysis for two days, because his mother had a slight cold. Knowing how great the boy's anxiety was, I then wrote to her urging her to send him if she possibly could. I thought his aunt might have been willing to bring him, if she knew his need. The mother herself, however, then brought him, in spite of her cold (it was over an hour's journey); but she let him know that I had urged his coming. He came into the analytic room in an apparently light-hearted way, smiling at me. But when I responded with a smile, he said, in grave reproach: "*Why* do you laugh?" He then broke the arm off a doll, and went on to break every toy in the room which, as later material showed, stood for the analyst and the father. He refused to co-operate with me, or have anything to do with me. Standing in a corner by himself, he talked in a deep cold voice, remote and detached, not to me, but apparently to himself (unconsciously to the internalized father), saying: "Yes, you *are* a cruel Daddy". It appeared that if I made his mother bring him to me when she was ill, this led to his projecting his internalized bad father on to me. I thus became a cruel father who could not be of any use to him, either. He then took a bowl of water and tried to pour it down his chest, inside his clothes. When I told him he wanted to punish his father and make him have a cold instead of his mother, so as to save his mother from him, Jack turned the water on to me, trying to pour it down my chest. Doubtless he feared that if his mother came out with him when she had a cold, she would have pneumonia as he himself had had, or tuberculosis like his father, and would die.

The interpretation of these fears about me as a bad external figure, and his anxieties about the cruel internalized father, relieved the boy's mind, so that he could leave in a calmer and more friendly state.

From this point, the analysis worked over more fully the various internal and external situations already described. I was able gradually to link the boy's feelings and phantasies to all these crucial happenings in the external world, and show him much of their meaning. The obsessional need to undress, and the compulsive urination on the floor, had already disappeared. The tantrums and excitement at home lessened considerably, and Jack became more amenable. The treatment was terminated by the mother earlier than I wished it to be, partly owing to the improvement, and partly because of a change of circumstances which made it still more difficult to bring the boy to me. (He had nearly five months' analysis in all.)

External Reality and Unconscious Phantasies

The various external happenings of the boy's life and all the details of his actual psychological environment had to be kept in mind throughout the analysis, and brought into relation with the phantasies expressed in his play, whenever Jack showed me that these events were active in his mind. And this applied not only to the crucial events of the period I have described, such as the accidents to mother and aunt and the grandmother's operation, but also to the general influence of the emotional relationships of mother and aunt and uncle, with the boy and with one another. As I have shown, the prudish and negative attitudes of the mother, calling his genital "rudy" and depreciating his manliness, affected the boy's own feelings and phantasies. They were an adverse influence, both in themselves and in what they revealed, to the sensitive eye of the boy, of the mother's own troubles. They contributed much to strengthen Jack's castration anxieties, and confirmed his feeling that his father's penis (both as represented by the external one of the uncle, and as internalized in himself), was harmful and disgusting; and that sexuality was a bad thing. In this way, his mother's feelings about sexuality made it harder for the boy to develop trust in his uncle or confidence in himself.

Above all other facts, however, the central underlying fact of the death of his father had to be brought into relation with the circumstances consequent upon it, as well as with the feelings and phantasies it aroused. As we have seen, the early loss of the father fostered all Jack's phantasies about the mysterious, sadistic and frightening qualities of the internalized father. Such internalization of the parents takes place with every child, as we know. The ordinary partings and apparent loss, the comings and goings, of the father and mother in the ordinary run of everyday life play an important part in the normal process of introjection. But in normal circumstances, the parents who go away from the child and seem to be lost constantly return and are rediscovered day by day and occasion by occasion. Thus, for the infant, seeing and talking to the father, having actual experience of him as an external figure, modify the phantastic quality of the internalized father as well, and render the internal figure less dominant in the mental life as a whole.

In Jack's case, the loss of his father had been absolute at a very early age. His relationship with his uncle as a substitute for his father had done much for him; but it had by no means fully modified in the boy's mind the dominant influence of the primitive and sadistic internalized father.

In the expression of his phantasies in play, Jack also made use of many details of real experience in everyday life, of a sort familiar to every child; e.g. he pretended that everything black or dirty or broken was "coal" and "carted it away". Here he used his everyday knowledge of coal, of what it is and what it does and what is done with it. He used his observations that "black stuff" can be useful and give us comfort, can be a pleasant sight when it is burning, in order to diminish his fear that fæces are altogether harmful and dangerous, and to increase his feeling that they are "good" and benign. That is to say, he used his perception of reality as a defence against anxiety and as a means of building up trust in his inner world.

Such universal threads in the actual experience of every child are part of the ready-to-hand material by means of which the ego builds itself up and strengthens certain of its defences. In the actual work of analysis, one has to regard such ordinary details of experience as having a vivid personal and emotional meaning, in the moment when they are used, as they needs must have when the child first discovers them. One has to be able to see the world through the eyes of the very young child, to understand that perception and reality-testing play an important part in the defences against anxiety which the ego employs. (N. Searl (1929) has drawn attention to the mechanism of the "flight to reality", and shown its operation in many important details.)

It is of vital importance to pay attention to the general conditions and the specific events in the patient's life, both present and past; but I shall now go on to emphasize the conclusion that none of these details of actual experience would carry us very far without knowledge of their precise meaning to the patient himself; in other words, without understanding of the unconscious phantasies which they stir up and foster, or help to neutralize, and the feelings and defences which are associated with these phantasies.

Take, for instance, the boy's first action in the analytic room, his putting the toy engine between two coaches and asking me "Engines *do* go like this, don't they? You *do* have a coach in front, don't you?" (As I have shown, some of the significance of this was clear to me, in relation to what I already knew of the boy's circumstances. But much more meaning was brought out in later sessions, since Jack often arranged the engine and coaches in the same way, in different analytic contexts.)

The boy knew quite well, of course, that engines, in actual practice, run in front of the coaches and not between them. Thus it was clear that, in his action and query, he denied a piece of knowledge in a symbolic way. In our experience, denial is primarily a defence against anxiety and an attempt to solve unconscious conflicts. What the boy was concerned with was the abnormal situation at home, where one man, his uncle, was between two women, and they were treated in an unequal way by him. Furthermore, this play expressed his protest against his mother's claim that "ladies go first", and his doubt about her reliability and truthfulness. Unconsciously, he saw in this demand a sign of her depreciation of his manliness and of his wish for independence, ultimately a sign of her intention to castrate him. One source of this anxiety was his own desire to steal his uncle's penis, incorporating it orally and anally; and this turned his mother into a persecuting rival. Considering again the conditions in which he lived, "ladies first" also meant that his mother envied the privileged position of the aunt who was really the first lady in the house and came first with the uncle. This fact was of particular importance, because guilt and anxiety are always greatly reinforced if the object attacked in phantasy is unhappy in actual reality.

This brings us to another point of importance. Melanie Klein has found that, in her experience, the tendencies of the boy's inverted Œdipus complex are influenced in quantity and quality if there actually are two women in the father's life. The fact that reality shows that it is possible to dethrone the mother and rob her of the father's love acts as a constant stimulus to the boy's impulses to be her rival and his desires for the father. It gives him ground for the excuse that the mother proved incapable of satisfying the father; on the other hand, it shifts the feelings of rivalry from the mother to the other woman, the interloper, and blends the rivalry with the wish to rescue and avenge the mother. With Jack, the situation was still more complicated and bewildering, since whilst the uncle was actually the aunt's husband, he was yet Jack's father-substitute and should (in Jack's unconscious mind) have belonged to his mother. Thus a situation was created in which both mother and aunt were felt to be intruders, and he, by sleeping with the uncle, deprived and robbed both women. These various interpretations were made to the boy in the relevant contexts and at the appropriate time.

Take, again, the first detail of the boy's response to his aunt's accident: "I *must not* sing". Why must he not sing? He had often been told to be quiet, not sing or shout: and before the accident already knew that his shouting could make mother and aunt cross. But he had been singing when the accident occurred, and this proved to his mind that his singing was really destructive, as bad as his shouting, which made "people's faces black": at this point, therefore, singing became equated with his fæces, the destructiveness of which, as we know, was a particular source of anxiety to him.

This experience is worth while stressing as a fact of general importance. Inherent in ambivalence is the uncertainty as to whether feelings of love or feelings of hate will prevail: ultimately whether the life or the death instinct will predominate. This means that the object of love is felt to be in a precarious state; the haunting question is: can mother (or father) be saved, or will she be destroyed? This doubt may expand and extend from one person to all people, both in the external and the internal worlds. (And, as Freud (1909) has pointed out, to doubt our own capacity to love leads us to doubt everything.)

The subject's feelings about the security or insecurity of those whom he loves—and hence the security of his own life—are determined in part by the degree of his ambivalence. In this struggle between love and hate external events often decide the issue. With Jack, his aunt's accident proved to him that his singing did not (as it had seemed to him to do) express friendly and cheerful feelings, but rather a malign and destructive influence. If we weigh the importance of external against internal factors, we could say that there might have been no outbreak of acute psychotic anxieties in Jack during these weeks, if the series of traumatic events had not occurred; but it would be equally true to say that if (for various reasons) he had had more trust in his love feelings and his internal world, he would have been able to withstand the impact of these events to a greater extent. As it happened, the aunt's fall had a far-reaching effect which involved his feelings about all his family. We must remember that, at the time of the aunt's accident, the operation on his grandmother's eyes was already pending, and had been frequently discussed in the boy's presence. There was no doubt that it weighed much on his mind and caused anxieties and conflicts. In his phantasy, his aunt's fall was an evil portent for his grandmother's operation; if his singing was destructive to the one, it would harm the other as well. (It will be remembered that Jack vividly expressed the deep feeling that he should "weep his eyes out for Granny".)

When, therefore, the boy said to me "I *must not* sing", he was not only repeating an external prohibition, important though this was; he was also expressing his feeling that his mother and aunt and grandmother *needed* from him that he should "weep his eyes out", and feel sorrow and grief for their suffering. But to "weep his eyes out" meant both to suffer blindness and to be castrated. He felt he *should* endure this, in order to save his grandmother and aunt pain and injuries. But such a demand, from himself or from others, could only bring the acme of anxiety and despair. As he showed me later on in his play, when he could not bear to assume the part of the grandmother ill in bed but had to make me do it instead, he *could not* accept this rôle, because it meant castration. Castration meant not only loss of his genital and renunciation of all libidinal gratification, but also giving up hope of creativeness in every sense, including the greatest and most important means of reparation.

After telling me, therefore, "I *must not* sing", he had instantly to deny this internal demand, acting out his aggression in a defiant way, throwing water about and flooding the floor, re-enacting the crash of his aunt's fall, with bravado and exaggerated enjoyment. If he cannot have the good penis and has no hope of saving his aunt and grandmother without suffering the extreme penalty himself, then the only thing left is to enjoy having a bad penis, to act out both his own aggression and that of the internalized bad father. But a few moments later, guilt again overcame him, and then he had to project the bad father and his own aggressive impulses on to me, reproach me with wearing a new frock when his aunt was hurt and unhappy, and throw wet rags at me to punish and spoil me.

The consideration of the meaning of this one fragment "I *must not* sing" (a meaning which unfolded itself gradually, and could only be understood in the whole context of circumstances and phantasy) has thus led us to note (*a*) the way in which actual experiences and psychical reality are all the time intimately interwoven; and (*b*) the relation between different defence mechanisms, and the way in which one gives place to another, whether under the onslaught of circumstances, or in response to interpretation and the shift of inner strains and stresses which interpretation brings about.

Main Anxieties

Let us now summarize the main anxieties of the patient.

(*a*) *Œdipus complex*

When Jack began his analysis, his direct Œdipus wishes were strongly repressed and overlaid by his dependence upon his uncle and the inverted Œdipus trends. I have shown how my interpretations of the more obvious meanings of his first doubting question to me (about the engine and coaches), in especial his fear of his mother as a castrator, brought some relief and a strong positive transference, releasing his heterosexual desires. Repression was lifted to some degree, and the Œdipus complex began to come into the open, including the anxieties of castration by the uncle.

At various points ensuing in the analysis, whenever Jack's anxieties were relieved by the interpretations, his direct heterosexual wishes appeared again. It will be remembered, for instance, how he asked me to show him my "leg and knees", after some of his anxieties about his own flatus and fæces had been relieved and his feelings of guilt and responsibility towards his internalized parents (father and grandmother) and his wish to revive his father and restore his grandmother had been admitted.

I have also shown how the special circumstances of Jack's life contributed to his using his homosexual attachment and sub-missive feminine wishes towards his uncle as a defence against all the dangers attaching to the Œdipus complex. His emotional dependence upon his uncle would in his situation inevitably have been very strong. He might, however, have been more able to sublimate his homosexual desires and identify himself more fully with his uncle, as a friendly helper in the external world, if his anxieties about the dead internalized father had not been so great. It was these depressive anxieties which kept him sub-jected to his bodily wishes towards his uncle—these bringing their own acute fears in their turn. He needed so intensely to obtain and incorporate (orally and anally) his uncle's penis, in order to counteract and overcome his dread of the dead father within him. The earliest oral and anal wishes were thus once again operative towards his uncle, with all their attendant anxieties. The lessening of these depressive anxieties in the course of the analysis led to a greater belief in the possibility of incorporat-ing a good penis and of restoring the actual mother, giving her life and babies by means of his own genital. The boy's homo-sexual wishes were to a greater extent sublimated, and his actual relation with his uncle thereby improved whilst at the same time he could more easily tolerate the anxieties relating to his hetero-sexual genital aims.

(b) Castration fears

Jack's castration anxieties were acute and were shown in a variety of ways (e.g. his putting the long line of trucks to represent my genital; his hitting his own head with a truck and falling down saying "Now I'm dead", after seeing his grandmother's bandaged head.)   Sometimes, when his direct Œdipus wishes towards his mother or myself were in the forefront, he feared castration by his uncle.   At other times, when the inverted Œdipus situation and his feminine wishes towards his uncle were predominant, it was the women, mother, aunt, myself, who would rob him of his penis, in jealous revenge. At still other times, both parties, the women and his uncle, became persecutors and castrators in his mind.   At such moments, his anxieties reached an extreme height, since then he had no good helping figure to whom he could turn for protection.

(c) Depressive anxieties

Marked as his castration fears were, however, the boy's

concern was very far from being only for himself and his own penis or body. He was also concerned about his mother and uncle and aunt. Even before he so plainly showed his grief and distress for his women-folk, he was often sad in mien and tone, when he was not being defiantly cheerful and omnipotent. His first anxious, doubting question at the beginning of his analysis already contained an element of grief and unhappiness. Many details of his play soon showed a deep underlying depression. This was, of course, most marked during the period of the crucial events; but it was there all the time, to a discerning eye. In the course of the analysis it became clear that unconsciously Jack mourned for his father, and longed to have him back, as a loved person, both for himself and his mother. He missed his guidance and protection, and felt that he himself ought to take his father's place in caring and providing for his mother, of whose unhappiness he was well aware.

That his anxiety and depression referred not only to the actual people in his external world, however, but also and primarily to his internalized objects, was shown in many details: e.g. his drawing of his father's face in the middle of the soapsuds, saying that the soapsuds were his father's "tummy"; telling me it was his "own bad gas" which had "flared up and burnt" and killed his father; burning the bag (representing his own body) which had contained the soldiers; burning up quantities of paper, representing his father's burning penis; singing about "something inside which cannot be denied, which I cannot hide"; talking to himself (to his internalized father) in the remote way which took no account of my presence: "You *are* a cruel Daddy". In his sweeping of the chimney (representing his anus) with the broom, he showed how he wanted to incorporate a good penis in order to expel the bad one already there and equated with his own fæces. This was an expression of his longing for a good father— either his uncle or his own father come to life—a longing which was itself part of his depression.

This internal situation, in which he fears that his feelings of hate and aggression, and his own excrements, endanger his loved internal objects (his "bad gas" "flares up and kills" his father) and threaten all sources of good with destruction, is an essential aspect of the infantile depressive position. These early feelings and phantasies had been made active again by the series of distressing events, which seemed to deprive him of the reassurance and help which he so much needed from the external world, in order to overcome the dangers of his internal situation.

When these depressive anxieties were at their worst, the picture became one of suicide. Explicitly suicidal trends were shown in Jack's "shooting" himself and wanting me to "shoot him dead"; his lying under the hearth-rug and wanting me to walk upon him there; his lying naked and limp on the chest of drawers (which to him was like a coffin); his compulsive nakedness in the cold weather; his deliberate attempt to pour water down his chest and give himself a cold (like his mother) and pneumonia (which he had recently had).

These actively suicidal tendencies appeared in the analysis when it seemed to him that I was actually a bad person, not only to him but also to his mother; when I seemed to be a bad father who would not or could not help *her* but would smile at or gratify *him*. In other words, when he felt he could only get relief or help or pleasure, or become potent, at the expense of his mother. This was shown when he spoke to the "cruel Daddy" inside him, completely withdrawn from contact with me, and tried to pour the water down his chest—because I had (as he thought) persuaded his mother to bring him to the analysis when she herself was ill. He showed me clearly, too, that it sometimes seemed to him that the sequence of distressing events at home, happening whilst he was in analysis with me, had come about *as a result* of his analysis—in his unconscious phantasy, because I indulged and seduced him, encouraged his greedy, uncontrollable wishes and brought out all the bad things from inside him.

In these aspects of the transference situation, I represented the evil internalized father who was the true object of his suicidal attacks upon himself. It was this father who was so dirty that he must be called a "gutter urchin" and treated as one, who was so dangerous (to mother and to the boy himself) that he must be burnt up, shot dead, trampled upon, laid naked in the cold and altogether destroyed. Jack's suicidal wishes were unconsciously directed against this bad internalized father and father's penis.

(When the boy lay naked and limp on the chest of drawers, however, his erection showed that there was a masochistic, libidinal element in this situation of despair and death. His masochism and homosexual libidinal trends were shown in many other ways, too, as I have instanced. The function of the masochistic trends in the suicidal situation is a profound and complex question into which I cannot enter here.)

REGRESSION AND HALLUCINATION

Under the stress of all these acute anxieties, certain regressive tendencies in the boy's mental life appeared during the analysis. These regressive trends can be seen at work in many of the details quoted. They were in operation to some extent before the analysis, both in his symptoms and in his emotional relationships to his family; but they appeared most active at certain points in the analysis, especially when the "lions, tigers and walruses" were hallucinated.

On the libidinal side, there was a regression from the genital to the pregenital level, as certain elements in the play with burnt paper, the biting and "shooting", the references to "bad gas", the defæcating on the table, etc., made plain. As regards object-relationships, there was a regression from the less ambivalent feelings of the genital level, with the wish to give love and the effort to keep and restore his loved objects, to the sadism of the anal-urethral level, where hate predominates and the objects of desire become tormentors and persecutors. Furthermore, the phantasied objects themselves (actual persons) regressed to part-objects (parts of persons, fæces and urine).

The picture became one of marked paranoid fears, in which the boy feared for his own life, because of the phantasied attacks on his own inside by the dangerous objects there. The phantasies of omnipotence, when Jack felt that his singing had made his aunt fall and injure her wrist, were so marked that it appeared that his reality-sense was also to some degree regressively affected by his anxiety.

The regressive tendencies in Jack's mental life were, however, seen at their most acute in his hallucination of the "lions". This happened on two occasions, when I had either refused to let him undress or urged him strongly to put on his clothes again. His dread of his internal persecutors was so great that he was driven to get them out of himself by undressing and exhibiting his erect genital. My refusal deprived him of the only way in which at the moment (he felt) he could overcome his internal danger. I myself thus became an external persecutor, the internalized "lion-father" being projected on to me. But then he lost me as a helping external figure, and felt he was endangered from within and without. There were persecutors everywhere. It was at this point that the hallucination occurred. Perceptual reality-testing was overborne by the intensity of his anxieties, and an earlier mode of dealing with inner reality was re-instated. He saw the lions there, as perceptual objects. The dangerous internalized father was first projected on to me, and then hallucinated in the "lions, tigers and walruses".

This hallucination may thus be regarded as a regressive phenomenon having a defensive function, against acute persecutory anxieties. The loss of reality-sense was a measure of the boy's emotional stress at the time.

Let us now summarize other defences which the patient used against his impulses and anxieties, and which have been instanced in the quoted material.

CHARACTERISTIC DEFENCES

(a) Projection

We have seen how often Jack attempted to get rid of all his dangerous inner objects by projecting them in various ways. His bodily processes (urination and defæcation) were sometimes felt by him to be the means of disposing of his persecutors: e.g. when he defæcated in the lavatory and then felt so sure that I should let him undress, because he had got rid of the dirty and dangerous things from inside him. At other times, he acted this out in some symbolic play.

(b) Denial

Jack often denied his psychical reality in an omnipotent manner; e.g. in his loud shouting and defiant singing, his assertion that the bonfire was "lovely", his "swimming" in his urine, his blacking of his own body, his coming into the room in a blatantly care-free manner after his aunt's accident, and so on.

(c) Exhibiting

Jack's undressing and showing his erect genital were closely related to both these mechanisms of denial and projection. In part, as we have seen, taking his clothes off meant getting rid of the bad things from the inside; in part it meant denying that his genital was dangerous. It was also a defence against his castration fears. The libidinal pleasure, which going naked and showing his erect genital gave him, was used as a means of defence against all these anxieties.

(*d*) *Masturbating*

Much of Jack's play in the analysis was a symbolic masturbation. It is widely accepted that, among other functions, masturbation is a defence against anxiety. With Jack, it was a defence against depressive anxieties, as well as castration fears. For instance, it became clear to me early in the analysis, when Jack made "Pluto" dance and "jig about", that this not only represented masturbation, but also his phantasy of bringing his dead father to life again, and letting him have a good sexual intercourse with mother. Reparation tendencies, thus, also played a part in his masturbation.

(*e*) *Controlling*

Much of the time in the analysis, Jack showed his wish to control me, both as an external figure and as representing his inner objects. E.g. when he made me go out of the room first, whilst he shouted loudly at me. In his insistent undressing, too, Jack was controlling and defying me and his mother. In all the burning of paper, stamping the flames out, playing with the electric plug and fire, and many other details, there was this element of omnipotent control.

REPARATION AND SUBLIMATION

The working out of Jack's aggression and libidinal wishes in play during the analysis, together with the interpretations (i.e. the expression in words of the secret wishes and fears and phantasies) gradually increased his feeling that it could be a good thing to bring secret things out into the open. The boy's guilt about deceiving those who loved him, by having secret greed and hate, secret dead things inside him, was to some extent relieved; and this helped him to feel that he might have good objects and loving people inside him. His compulsion to project what was inside, coming up in the analysis, especially after the crucial happenings in his home, gives us a hint of the great efforts which Jack had hitherto made to keep the secret evil hidden inside. His easy friendliness and rather defiant cheerfulness, before the analysis, had covered up a considerable depression. All the greater was his relief, when repression was to some extent lifted, at being able to bring things out in the analysis. By this process, his libido was freed and felt to be a support to his ego. This change was interrupted for a time by the severe strain of the traumatic events, which threw the boy back to his early psychotic anxieties.

After these acute anxieties were worked through and analysed, there was, as I have said, much improvement in Jack's difficulties at home, and a steady progress in the analysis itself. He began to feel more confidence in his reparation aims, and there were signs of development towards the sublimation of his libidinal desires. (I have found that these two processes, reparation and sublimation, are always mutually dependent.)

Jack's reparation wishes were shown in many details of the analysis. It will be remembered that he felt his excrements to be extremely dangerous and destructive to other people. His efforts to keep or make things clean (e.g. in putting a towel representing a baby's napkin on the seat of the chair, washing the walls and the floor representing "Granny's bottom" and "Daddy's tummy", sweeping the chimney clean, etc.) must therefore be looked upon as true reparation, which could not be adequately described as "reaction-formation". These activities meant much more than being clean; they were ways of keeping his grandmother alive and reviving his dead father. They were bound up with his love and his feelings of guilt towards these loved people. Other instances of reparation were his feeding the toy babies, being the "sailor saving the babies" from drowning, giving me (his grand-mother) "tea" to drink and little toys to comfort me when I was "ill in bed", making the dolls in the basin of water (representing the good parents inside himself) have a good intercourse ("they're cuddling each other"), writing and drawing on the table, for the first time, immediately after defæcating there.

Meaning of Symptoms

Jack had made very great efforts to adapt to his restrictive environment, to win the love of his family and keep them happy; hence his "easy" friendliness and enforced cheerfulness, occasion-ally tinged with sadness and unhappiness. His relatively normal general state, apart from his specific symptoms, before the analysis, was however a deceptive condition. His depressive anxieties were to a large extent dissociated from the ordinary current of his mental life, and found their only outlet in his two chief symptoms, his violent tantrums and his moments of "queer" excitement.

I did not see his tantrums in their full violence in the analysis. Jack's anger and obstinacy when I would not let him undress came nearest to his behaviour at home and school, but interpretation prevented the anxiety expressed in the tantrums from reaching its full height. The phantasies underlying the tantrums appeared in a less condensed form in much of Jack's play and many of the analytic situations. E.g. in his attacks upon the evil, castrating, internalized father, burning him, "shooting" him dead, trampling on him, etc., Jack showed me how, in his tantrums, he was fighting and defying the dangerous father and father's penis inside him, projected on to an external authority. In his tantrums, when he was frustrated by his environment, the boy screamed and shouted louder than his internal father, kicked and bit him, proved himself the stronger, and defied all external compulsions and threats as well.[1]

At times of somewhat less acute anxiety, moments of libidinal excitement, the boy enacted his possession of a good live internal penis—or, rather, his possession *by* such a penis—in his "fits" of intense excitement, the excitement which was not anger, but was described as "queer" and uncontrolled. Again, I did not see these "fits" in the analysis, since the over-determined material which lay behind them was brought out in a less condensed and dissociated form. His doubts about the goodness of this internal penis remained and were, in my view, responsible for the "queerness" and detachment, the dissociation of his excitement. He had to detach himself from his external world, partly in order not to endanger the external sources of good; but partly, also, not to be robbed of the pleasure which his "fits" contained, as an expression of the phantasy of a good internal penis, kept secretly inside himself, with sexual feeling.

The psychic content of his "fits" was entirely repressed. These "fits" of queer excitement, represented in the analysis, e.g. in "Pluto's" dancing about, expressed both his libidinal wishes and his desire to revive his dead father. They were linked with his unconscious masturbation phantasies, and were in part a substitute for masturbation, a defence against it.

*   *   *   *   *

In conclusion, I wish to say again that the study of this case

---

[1] In a former paper (1940) I described other cases in which these unmanageable anxieties about dangerous and frustrating internal objects were dealt with in temper tantrums, and considered the subject generally.

(*a*) shows how intimately external and internal reality are intertwined in the symptoms, the developmental history and the analytic responses of an individual; and

(*b*) what serious difficulties may be masked by a general appearance of reasonable normality, in a patient whose symptoms might easily be considered normal for early phases of childhood (the temper tantrums), or relatively unimportant in the whole picture he presents (the "queer" excitement).

REFERENCES

ABRAHAM, K. (1924). (*Trans.* 1927.) "A Short Study of the Development of the Libido," *Selected Papers*, 418.

FREUD, S. (1909). (*Trans.* 1925.) "Notes upon a Case of Obsessional Neurosis," *Collected Papers*, III, 376.

— (1917). (*Trans.* 1925.) "Mourning and Melancholia " *Collected Papers*, IV, 158.

— (1923). (*Trans.* 1927.) *The Ego and the Id.*

GLOVER, E. (1932). "A Psycho-Analytic Approach to the Classification of Mental Disorders," *J. Ment. Sci.*, *78*, 819.

HEIMANN, P. (1942). "A Contribution to the Problem of Sublimation," *Int. J. Psycho-Anal.*, *23*, 8.

ISAACS, S. (1940). "Temper Tantrums in Early Childhood," *Int. J. Psycho-Anal.*, *21*, 280.

KLEIN, M. (1929). "Infantile Anxiety-Situations Reflected in a Work of Art," *Int. J. Psycho-Anal.*, *10*, 436.

— (1932.) *The Psycho-Analysis of Children.*

— (1935). "A Contribution to the Psychogenesis of Manic-Depressive States," *Int. J. Psycho-Anal.*, *16*, 145.

RIVIERE, J. (1936). "A Contribution to the Analysis of the Negative Therapeutic Reaction," *Int. J. Psycho-Anal.*, *17*, 304.

SEARL, N. (1929). "The Flight to Reality," *Int. J. Psycho-Anal.*, *10*, 280.

XII

FATHERLESS CHILDREN[1]

(1945)

THE presence of a wise and affectionate father gives to the child a sense of security in his life, a control upon which he can rest and within which he can adventure, an ideal towards which he can hopefully strive. When father and mother are loving and united in the home, the child can reach out to independence and a life of his own, and yet keep an intimate awareness of mutual affection and mutual need.

No one could read Miss Sharpe's[2] description of the healthily developing child, in the happy possession of both parents, without feeling a painful sense of the sad fate of so many children to-day. For vast numbers of children, the loss of the father is added to all the strain, confusion and suffering of war, of ruined homes and divided families. The foundations of life have been uprooted, and society destroyed. Little is left that is secure and good in their worlds.

How important it is for those who seek to help these bereaved and bewildered children, to know what such a loss amid the terrible upheaval of the world means to the *minds* of the children! Difficult as may be the task of supplying food, cleanliness and medical care to the fatherless and homeless children of Europe to-day, it is simple when compared with the educational and psychological problem. To help these children overcome the evil effects of the last six years requires a deep knowledge of what six years of war and the spectacle of a world in ruins may do to their feelings and their ideals. We cannot find how to help them without such understanding.

In this booklet, however, we are considering in particular what the death of a father may mean to his children, whether in peace or war. Even when the background of life remains secure, the loss of the father's affectionate guidance may lead to far-reaching

---

[1] From *Fatherless Children*, N.E.F. Monograph No 2 edited by Peggy Volkov, M.A., Ph.D.
[2] Op. cit. *What the Father Means to a Child*.

changes in the child's emotional development and in his attitudes to other people. In a later paper, Joan Riviere[1] shows what it means to a mother to lose her helpmeet and the father of her children. Here we shall speak of what it means to the children to lose their father.

What it Means to Children when Their Father Dies

As Mrs. Riviere points out, the children's loss is in many ways greater than the wife's, since she has many resources to turn to in her adult life and character which they have not. The parents (father no less than mother) are unique and primary objects of love. All later loves (husband and wife as well as friends) are built upon these first ones and in large part are substitutes for them. Moreover, the children need the father not merely as someone to love, but also as a pattern and control in their development. They feel his loss in their inner life, as well as in their external dependence.

Even in the first year of life, before the child can speak, the disappearance of the father from his world awakens feelings of bewildered grief and stirs great anxiety in the child. We can see clear signs of such emotions in some children. Others are only able to show them indirectly, in less easily recognized forms. In many, they issue in symptoms of neurosis and difficulties of behaviour at a later age.

Here are two examples which show that even in his earliest days the child feels the death of the father acutely. A little girl, whose father was killed in the war just before her birth, began to ask questions about "Daddy" as soon as she could talk. (She is a highly intelligent child and spoke very early.) She was shown his photograph and called it "Daddy" and spoke to it and kissed it. But later on (at about two and a half years), she evidently compared the photo with the actual fathers of her playmates, and began to look for a *live* father herself. She now asked "Why doesn't he speak to me?" and "Why doesn't my Daddy come?" When she was told that "he had gone up in his bomber and could not come home", she asked, "Doesn't he want to come and see me?" We thus see how she longs, even at so young an age, to have a real live father who will talk to her and respond to her. She shows, too, how puzzled she is at his not coming and how ready to

[1] Op. cit. *The Bereaved Wife.*

feel that "he doesn't *want* to come". In other words, she fears that his not coming means that he does not love her.

A second instance is of a boy of four years whose moods of unhappiness and neurotic symptoms caused him to be brought to a psychologist for treatment. The boy was subject to severe tantrums and "queer fits" of excitement which the people around him could not understand. He was an affectionate and trusting child. In his treatment, the boy was encouraged to express his feelings and phantasies to the psycho-analyst by means of his dramatic play with various materials, and gradually the core of his difficulties was made plain. They centred round his tangle of feelings about his father's death and his mother's unhappy circumstances. His father had died in the first year of his life. The mother was poor and had to go out to earn her living in ways she did not like, whilst living with a sister and her husband. The boy showed that he felt great distress about his mother's loneliness and poverty, and the hard work she had to do. He resented his father's having died and felt he *ought* to be alive: he was a "bad Daddy" because he was not there to take care of the mother. In the primitive logic of the little child's imagination, the boy felt that if Daddy had been "good" he would have been alive and helpful. His love and sorrow for his mother made the boy long to help her and feel that he must take his father's place with her as a protector. This was naturally a great burden to so young a child, and it increased his resentment against his father for not being there to help. The boy longed for his father for his own sake, too, as someone to love, someone to help and guide him, someone to show him how to become a father himself. And he came to feel intensely guilty and responsible for his father's death, because of his own early rivalry with him for mother's love. It seemed to the boy (again in the primitive logic of the child's imagination) that it was *his* fault that father had died; his own hostile wishes had killed him. This was shown very plainly in his play with the analyst, and even expressed spontaneously in words. Such feelings of guilt and resentment made it very hard for the boy to believe in the power of his own love and good wishes or in his own future as a man and as a father. These and other complex feelings struggled within the boy and found their outcome in his moods of sadness and his neurotic symptoms.

The father's absence and death affects the children's lives in many actual and concrete ways as well. The younger children (and sometimes the older ones as well) suffer from the sense that they have lost a protector. They feel that father is not there to keep them safe from real dangers—the risks of crossing the road or travelling on the train, from thunder and lightning, fire and bombs, from not having a comfortable home to live in, with good things to enjoy, from not having enough to eat and wear. They miss this sense of actual bodily security which the father's nearness gives them, as well as their belief that he will be there to help them in the crises of later life, such as choosing their occupation and getting trained for it. The actual loss of support and protection contributes greatly to the child's sense of insecurity and dread of the future, after the father's death.

The two examples already noted show us how great the effect of losing the father in very early life—even in the first year—may be. The event causes intense conflict of feeling, pain and grief, fear and guilt to the child of any age. But, contrary to what many people take for granted, the younger the child the more serious and far-reaching the influence of such a loss. The outward results of this conflict of intense feeling and of the way in which the child's imagination works upon his experience vary a good deal according to the age, the temperament, the previous mental balance or neurotic tendencies, and the particular circumstances of the children at the time.

In young children who lose their fathers, the moods and attitudes in which conflicting feelings are expressed may change from day to day or week to week, as the child tries now one way, now another, of overcoming his stress of feeling. Even in the middle years, when children are normally more stable, their moods may now change so rapidly that we never "know how to take them". Or they may behave in "odd" ways which surprise and puzzle those around. These changes in mood and behaviour and "odd" manners are often very trying to the grown-ups in the home or the school. They would puzzle and bother us less if we did not so often automatically deny the reality of the child's sense of loss and of his suffering. As Mrs. Riviere points out,[1] we are inclined to assume that children are "too young to realize". Our examples will have shown that even before the end of the first year, children are not "too young to realize" the fact of loss, and to be aware of a deep conflict of feeling about father's disappearance. They may be too young to *understand* the event, but that

[1] Op. cit.

only makes their suffering more acute. We should not be misled by the fact that children cannot as a rule explain in words what is going on in their minds. What they try to do is to control and master painful and frightening feelings by various forms of behaviour or various attitudes of mind.

Many young children become extremely spoilt after the father's death, clinging to the mother and tyrannizing over her in endless ways. The slightly older child may show open resentment against the mother whilst yet clinging to her, not with affection but peevishly and tyrannically. They are unable to part from mother and yet unable to be happy with her. Such tyrannical clinging arises from great anxiety on behalf of the mother. The fear of losing her as he has lost his father is genuine, but equally strong is the child's fear of his own destructiveness and possessiveness, and his guilt towards her because of his father's death. He feels *he* has turned father out and destroyed him and therefore his mother cannot now love him, the child. The girl may feel this, too, in the depths of her mind, since she loved her mother best in her very earliest days, and father was at first a rival for her mother's care. The constant demand for love and for his mother's presence arises from the child's need to be reassured against his fears that she has been hurt by him, or that she will cease to love him because of father's death. (Such excessive clinging to persons we love is always a sign of guilt towards them and anxiety about them. If love is more assured it does not need to cling so convulsively.)

Sometimes the bereaved children become rebellious and defiant, getting quite out of the mother's control. At school they may become very aggressive to other children, inclined to bully and torment those younger than themselves, as well as challenging and hostile to everyone in authority. Such conduct readily develops into seriously anti-social behaviour outside the school. In such delinquency, forever defying the law and trying to circumvent the teacher or the policeman, the child seems to be searching for someone powerful enough to control him and to condemn him for wrong-doing. He is, in other words, seeking his lost father, not so much as someone who will love and guide him, but rather as a just judge to punish and imprison him. The delinquent child tries, too, to get rid of his feeling of guilt by making others responsible for controlling his destructive impulses.

Early bereavement (whether the loss of father or mother) has been shown to be a frequent influence in a later developing tendency to anti-social behaviour, especially stealing. And thieving may break out immediately after the father's death.

Some fatherless children seem to search for the lost father by generally irresponsible behaviour, a tendency to defy convention and behave in a "Bohemian" way, to play truant and wander about the town or countryside, or to cast off friends and constantly seek new ones. In these cases, there seems to be more wish to find a friendly and loving father but little hope of doing so.

Other children become very lazy in work or lose all interest in normal pleasures and in social life, or turn away from all responsibility, to the point of extreme indifference and apathy. Still others try to deal with their feelings by becoming over-cheerful and boisterous in a way which can easily mislead the grown-ups into believing that they have no sense of loss or are incapable of suffering. (Such overcheerfulness and boisterous good spirits are often welcomed by the grown-ups because they do not cause much practical difficulty.) Some children, however, may put on a hard brightness which prevents any real contact with other people. This is a powerful denial of love and dependence, a defence against the dread of further loss and against painful feelings of guilt.

Another sort of hardness is shown by some who cannot bear to receive any sympathy or condolence or even kindness or consideration from the grown-ups in home or school. They cannot stand the slightest reference to their loss. It is as if their personal pride were involved or as if any recognition of the father's death by others implied a criticism or accusation against themselves. They refuse tender feelings because these seem to open the way to fear and guilt, which are intolerable.

This defence against painful feelings sometimes goes so far as to lead to a complete withdrawal of affection from everybody— mother, teacher, school fellows or friends. Such a state of mind is especially unfavourable for later development, since it means that the child has shut a door between himself and other people, and will thus be prevented from finding any substitutes for the lost father in later life or from enjoying the inner guidance which a loved and admired father figure can bring.

Such withdrawal of contact from other people and the denial of feeling sometimes lead to serious mental disease. It has, for example, been recorded in a recent investigation of schizophrenia (split personality) that a large proportion of patients suffering from this disease had experienced early bereavement.

Another mode of response to the tragic loss is acute depression. Here the child not only feels great sadness but also great unworthiness and self-reproach; in marked cases he loses belief in himself and any hope or ambition for the future. Yet this response is actually less ominous for the child's future than when he turns to delinquency or to a complete denial of feeling, since here the child is at least able to share his distress with other people, and to acknowledge the reality of his loss and of his inner world.

Not infrequently, one outcome of the intense conflict of feelings aroused in boy or girl by the father's death is to turn away from loving those of the opposite sex, and to seek the affection and approval only of those of the same sex. In the boy this is another way of seeking the lost father, one which denies and overcomes rivalry, hate and resentment against him, by over-stressing love, admiration and submission to him, and denying love and longing for the mother. In effect the boy says: "I have not wanted my mother for myself nor hated my father; it is father whom I love and long for, whom I admire and will obey". He turns from the mother partly also because she has become a frightening person through *her* loss and *her* need, and through the son's guilt towards her, so strongly stirred by father's death. The daughter, too, may become defensively attached and submissive to her mother, not being able to assert herself in any way, not daring to take any love away from mother for a future husband and children, not able to believe that the bereaved mother will ever allow her to have a husband and children of her own. Old feelings of rivalry with the mother for father's love, and hostility to her, are now buried and denied under love and devotion. Some degree of over-devotedness to the mother in children whose father has died is extremely common, at least for a time. If it is too much welcomed and exploited by the mother for her own reasons, it may permanently distort the development of the children and make it impossible for them to find normal sexual fulfilment and parenthood in later life.

These are some of the many and various ways in which the pain and loss, the anxiety and guilt stirred in the children by the death of the father are dealt with in their minds. Sometimes one of these natural and spontaneous defences against overwhelming and conflicting feelings may be developed to a marked degree.

The child then becomes a "case" of delinquency, of depression, of homosexuality, of schizophrenia. Far more often, bereaved children show a fluctuating mixture of such disturbances of development, though in a less degree. The more normal the child, the more likely he is to deal with his feelings in a variety of different ways, now one, now another, according to his age and situation. Some disturbance of development, some form of expression of emotional conflict there is bound to be for a period of time. We cannot prevent such attitudes arising. The child has to go through his mourning. If he cannot do so openly, then he will do so inwardly. If we wish to help him, we must not ourselves deny the reality of his loss and the truth of his feelings about it. We must aim at enabling him to find such an expression of his feelings and such a way of dealing with them as will keep alive his relationship with other people, his capacity to love them and feel with them, and his belief in his own future.

How Can We Help Fatherless Children?

Let us consider now what forms of help we can give to fatherless children.

In the first place, we must realize that the loss of the father cannot wholly be made good. As Mrs. Riviere points out, no psychologist and no humanitarian can remove the reality of the loss and suffering of the bereaved wife. She has to mourn and only time can help her to make the needed inner re-adjustment. This is true of the children too. The loss of the father is a real fact, and no substitute, no external help, can altogether make up for him. All we can hope to do, with the utmost of our goodwill and understanding, is to help the child to accept that loss and find his way out of the conflict of feeling it arouses. Moreover, the child has to find his *own* way out. Just as children show their difficulties in different ways, so they will find different ways of overcoming them, whatever sort of help we give. We cannot determine the ultimate effect of his experience upon the child's character and social attitudes. We cannot say that his development shall take this line rather than that, nor decide what sort of person he shall become in the end. We can to some degree and in some form give him the support he looks for from the outer world, and the opportunities he so much needs to express his feelings and receive understanding.

The problem of helping children in this crisis of life has to be met both in the home and in the school and social life generally. We may discuss these separately. (In practice, however, the need for home and school to co-operate is even more urgent than with children who have their fathers to guide them.)

The Bereaved Child at Home

It will be seen from our chapter on the bereaved wife that the mother herself needs help from the outside world in dealing with the difficulties of the children. She needs support from her friends and the comforts of social life. She needs, if not immediately, then later on, some recreation and satisfaction outside the home. She needs help in understanding what is going on in the minds of the children and the opportunity to talk over their problems with other mothers in similar circumstances and with the children's teachers. If she has no specially wise friends, skilled social workers may be able to help her understanding of the children's development and needs.

The specific help she herself can give to her children depends partly upon their ages. She looms larger in the lives of the youngest children than in those of school age, and her influence is greater. With the younger members of the family, the whole burden of helping them rests upon her. The older ones will have their school fellows and teachers, or their companions at their clubs, to brace and reassure them.

The first thing is for the mother to realize that the children do have acute feelings of distress, of loss, of grief, of guilt and anxiety, and to allow them to express these feelings in whatever way they can.

The mother reveals her own attitude not only in words and open talk. The children, even the very young ones, *see* when their unhappiness is unwelcome to mother. They know by her manner and mood, or by what is *not* said, when she implicitly demands that they should have no feelings at all, but go on "as if nothing had happened". They are aware of it when their being more anxious, more frightened, more clinging and appealing, makes mother herself anxious or hostile. They may react to her demand that they should not show troublesome feelings by doing what she wants, denying their feelings and becoming polite automata. They may do the opposite thing and become still more whining and peevish, more dependent upon her, or else more rebellious.

But however they respond, they *know* when mother cannot allow them to mourn for father, when she resents their having any feeling about him and claims for herself all the sorrow and despair. They know, too, when she denies any deep sorrow and anxiety of her own and endeavours in an artificial way to "go on just the same" and to keep the family life undisturbed by this critical event. By such artificial composure in herself, she sets a premium upon falsity in them. They know she is refusing to admit real events as well as denying feelings.

Here is an example of the effects of such denial, harmful even when it springs from good motives: an intelligent boy of two and a half years had a devoted nurse who was knocked down and seriously injured by a car. The boy did not see the accident. His parents, knowing the affection the child had for his nurse and doubting her recovery, told the boy she had gone away for a holiday and evaded his questions or gave him reassurances when he asked why she did not come back. After some weeks they observed a marked change in his emotional attitude to them and to life in general. He developed an artificial way of speaking and a flippant manner in every situation, along with hints of distrusting his father and mother and being withdrawn from them. It was as if a mask of supercilious politeness were laid over the spontaneous nature of the boy. After a time his parents came to the conclusion that he had, in spite of all their care, sensed that something serious had happened to his nurse, that she was not just away on a holiday, but might never come back to him, and that his parents were pretending to him that all was well. Seeing this adverse development in the boy, the mother now told him the truth of what had happened, together with the reasons why she had not given him the truth before. The child's relief was at once very great, and he quickly returned to his normal spontaneity of feeling, of trust in his parents and intimacy with them.

Another example of the ill effects of the constant denial of suffering and emotional conflict on the part of the parents is of an adolescent girl, whose social manner was one of superficial ease, cheerfulness and serenity. But there was a lack of depth in her contact with people, and little capacity to appreciate or allow strong feelings in others. She gave an impression of shallowness and unreality, as if there were merely a shiny surface with little or nothing behind it. This character had been developed under the influence of her mother's way of dealing with the death of the father and of a twin sister. The mother had never allowed her own sufferings to appear openly to the children, never shared her cares with them, and in general had set before them an ideal of perfect control, perfect calm and reasonableness in every situation, no matter how grievous it might be. In the psycho-analytic treatment of the girl, it became clear that she had felt that her mother's attitude deprived her of real love. Her mother had pushed the daughter out of her inner life and refused to share true feelings with her. In her own phantasies the girl felt that this was because she herself was too mean, too jealous and hostile to be allowed to have any part in the mother's sorrow for her husband and other daughter. It made the girl permanently guilty and self-distrustful.

Such denial of feeling is something very different from its control and moderation. Children need both to be allowed to express their own feelings in whatever way they can find, and to have some share in mother's feelings too. It is best of all if feeling can be put into words, if mother and children, even the little ones, can speak of their sorrow and grief to each other. This is the safe way to learn to control and moderate feeling.

On the other hand it is not a good thing for the mother to *demand* expressions of sorrow and sadness from the children. It is not good if she forces outward signs of mourning upon them, will not allow them to be happy at any time, to play or seek the society of their friends, to take up again any of their ordinary pursuits. In any case, the children feel guilty about having a life of their own if father is dead. Their guilt should not be reinforced and strengthened by mother's demands or by her resentment against their wishes. To talk together of father, to revive memories of experiences shared with him in the family life, to remember together what he was like, what he did and said, to keep his photographs about, and in general to keep his image alive in the minds of the children is a good thing. But this, too, can be overdone. The mother should not *demand* of the children that they remember father and talk about him; she should be able to respond to their need to speak of him if they show it. Father's memory should be neither a forbidden nor too sacred a thing. It should be shared and share-able, warm and alive.

The younger children are likely to want to talk of father more freely than the adolescent boy or girl. The little ones will ask questions about what Daddy was like and what he said and did, and compare him with the fathers of their playmates. Most boys and girls in their teens are likely to be rather reserved; but there will be times, perhaps on a holiday or when some particular topic of meal-time talk comes up, one which links with father, when they will be able to bear to open their hearts again, share their memories once more with mother and ask questions about father. If she can receive these moments of confidence without demanding them, she can be of great help to her children.

The work of mourning has always a double aspect: on the one hand a keeping alive of the lost loved one in the mourner's mind by reviving memories, reliving experiences, feeling sorrow and love again; on the other, a giving up of the lost object of love and a turning to new persons. The children need to feel that both these things are possible, that in order to go forward in their own lives they do not have to destroy father altogether in their minds by denying their memories or what they have felt for him; nor that they have to put the whole of their love and mental energy into the effort of keeping him alive in their minds, thus being unable to turn to other people and other interests in the outside world.

The memory of the father, moreover, should not be treated as too holy or sacrosanct. Father should not be canonized or spoken of as someone who never could be criticized, one who had no faults. "That's not the way to speak of your father when he is dead". Such idealization of the dead parent has many disadvantages. It brings a sense of falsity and unreality. The children know that mother and they are conspiring to create an unreal picture. And the idealized father for whom mother allows nothing but reverence is of little use in the life of the children, and may even be harmful. The boy feels that mother looks upon father as someone so wonderful and perfect that he, the boy, could never attain to such heights. This perfect image of father which mother wants him to retain in his mind will act as a brake upon all the boy's own hopes and ambitions in the actual world. By inhibiting all normal criticism of adults, it may check his relationship with real men—friends, teachers, relatives—who could otherwise help to guide him and become a pattern for him in his further development. It may shut down on his school work and his ambitions for a career of his own, or prevent him from marrying and becoming a father himself.

The girl, too, may carry this idealized image of the perfect father so vividly in her mind that she measures every real man and possible husband by this unreal standard, and may never be able to find the husband she wants. Or it may lead her to feel that fathers are such wonderful beings that she herself could never be fit for a mate; and this attitude may rob her of normal fulfilment in marriage and motherhood.

A special point in time of war is the unwisdom of talking too much to the fatherless boy (especially if he is very young) of what a hero his father had been, how he died for his country as a soldier, and how the boy is expected to grow up and be such a hero too. In the depths of his mind, the young boy may hate his father for dying, for serving his country instead of looking after his family. The boy may become terrified of growing up, because that will (to him) mean being a soldier and giving up his own life—since it seems that that is what fathers do and are expected to do. Such a notion may lead to severe emotional conflict and most unsatisfactory development.

Another way in which the mother can help her bereaved children, both the little ones and the adolescents, is to bring them into contact with men who may become substitutes (as far as anyone ever can be) for the lost father. Male relatives, grandfathers, uncles, friends, even lodgers or older boy friends, can all be a great help to the children and, by renewing their emotional ties to a father figure, can lessen their sense of isolation and of exclusive dependence upon the mother. If they find other men to respect and love, this will give them some measure of external guidance and a pattern for them to follow, as well as strengthening the elements in their own internal life, which represent the guiding and controlling father. And if the mother herself can have friendly contact with men relatives or visitors, this, too, is a reassurance to the children. They then feel that she is not entirely deserted and alone in the world, wholly dependent upon them for help and affection. They feel free to be normally jealous once more. If through excessive devotion to the memory of her husband or her fear of being accused of disloyalty, the mother should deprive the children of social contacts and intimate friendships with other men, she is indeed doing them a disservice.

The children's love for their mother (and this applies to both boys and girls) will often lead them to offer her more practical help in the home after father's death. The girl as well as the boy may feel that they should try to take father's place and protect, cherish and serve mother more fully and freely than when father was alive. It is good that they should be allowed to help and to develop a sense of responsibility for the mother and for the home. To be able to do more for the mother reassures them against their anxiety and guilt towards her and father. It is, however, a fatal thing for their development if mother exploits this wish to help and demands too much from the children in practical ways or in devotedness. If she tries to comfort herself by retaining their services to the exclusion of outside interests and friendships or independent pursuits in the home, she may hamper their development permanently and turn their love into hidden hate. They will fear and distrust her and in the end she will have less happiness in her relationship with them.

Sometimes the mother is so placed—if she has a large family or has to go out to work—that she cannot avoid making big demands on the eldest boy or girl for practical help in the home—sharing the housework, mothering the younger children, running errands. But it is one thing to do this because it is necessary, as the children can understand, and another to do it because she wants them not to have lives of their own, not to enjoy themselves out of her ken. Her own attitude will be different according to these motives. In the first case she will let them off such tasks whenever she can, and will let the children feel that they are doing something for their own future as well as for her. It will be comradely and a real sharing. In the second, she will be possessive and grudging, and at bottom she will not appreciate what they do. And this will make all the difference to her children.

Again, the mother should not encourage a child of either sex to take father's place in her bed and sleep with her. Both boy and girl will often seek this, especially in the first days after father's death. They seek it in order to comfort both themselves and mother. To be able to take father's place with mother in this concrete way is, moreover, a fulfilment of the early wishes of the children, when they wanted to turn father out and possess mother altogether. It is partly because it fulfils these wishes that sleeping in mother's bed gives rise to anxiety and guilt on the part of the child; and the more guilty he is about having in phantasy turned his father out, the more anxious about the need to make up to mother for the loss of father, the more eagerly and persistently will he seek this reassurance of intimate bodily contact; and the more guilty and anxious will he then become. The situation becomes a vicious circle in which it is increasingly difficult for the child (whether boy or girl) to get free of this unwise intimacy and mutual dependence.

For the mother to indulge herself and the children in this way is undesirable even when the children are young. It becomes seriously harmful when boy or girl is approaching adolescence. There is a serious risk that the children may become permanently tied to the mother's needs, unable to grow up in their own feelings. Many a son whose father has died early becomes a bachelor, and, under cover of excessive devotion to his mother, develops deep hatred and distrust of her because he feels she has robbed him of his manhood.

In a typical example, a boy of ten or eleven years was encouraged to sleep with his mother after father's death in order to comfort her. He developed marked girlish characteristics (crying and blushing easily, being shy among adults, clinging to his mother); and he became inhibited in his school work and unable to achieve what was expected from him in view of his intelligence and previous character.

Once such a situation is brought about, moreover, the mother often finds it increasingly difficult to take the step of turning the boy out of her bed, since she imagines he will (as he may) take this as a serious rebuff and will never forgive her. It is far better never to begin the practice.

An instance of grave disturbance due to the same mistake, but at an earlier age, is of a young man of twenty, who came for psychoanalytic treatment because of his great fear of his exclusive concern with men and complete lack of interest in girls or women. Along with this went increasingly hostile feelings towards his mother, which distressed both of them. On the surface he was a devoted and admiring son, but he found himself more and more often overcome by gusts of violent irritation and less and less able to talk to her frankly and intimately. On the other hand, his longings for an intimate relation with men, his love and admiration for them, were very intense. He spoke of a particular man friend in the romantic and idealizing way in which most boys would speak of the first girl with whom they fell in love. At the same time he had impulses of cruelty towards the young men he was drawn to, with phantasies of hurting them and triumphing over them.   The outlook for his future seemed gravely unsatisfactory.

The young man's parents had separated when the boy was under two years of age, and the father had died not long after. The mother had turned to the boy to satisfy her longing for affection, and when he was still very young she talked to him almost as if he were grown up and demanded his exclusive devotion. He shared her room from his early days and throughout boyhood. Even after he went to a boarding school he still shared her room in the holidays. Her demand that he should hate his father and join with her against his memory was quite open and unlimited. The boy had given her a great love and had done his best to take his father's place, but the accumulated feelings of resentment against his mother for making these inordinate demands upon him and keeping him dependent upon her had led him secretly to idealize his father in his mind. Everywhere he looked for a father whom he could love. But it was an *ideal* father he sought, and each of his actual men teachers or friends in turn disappointed him. His secret hate and resentment against his mother prevented him from turning to other women as objects of love, since he feared that any affection towards another woman would always carry with it this hidden but intense fear and hatred as well. The love he might have given to another woman could never be withdrawn from his mother in the least degree. It had to be kept fixed on her because it was so much needed to overcome his fear and hatred of her. This young man was an extreme example of the ill effect upon the developing boy of excessive demands from the mother that he should devote himself entirely to her in order to fill the void left by his father. Too early and too strong a demand that the boy should take the father's place may thus in the end make it impossible for him ever to feel himself a father or to become so in actuality.

This demand by the mother upon the fatherless boy often goes along with excessive indulgence in various ways. He gets the sense that he can do what he likes with his mother; she is "soft" and cannot control him. Whatever she may say at first, she gives way to him in the end, and if he wheedles long enough or is obstinate enough, he can get all he asks for. This situation causes great anxiety in the depths of the boy's mind and is most unfavourable to his development. The mother needs to be firm and steady, no less than patient and loving, in her handling of the fatherless boy.

As already suggested, mothers can help their bereaved boys and girls by encouraging their friendships with other children and their recreation and social life outside the home. If they join with other friends in sport and games and social activities they will actually love her the better, and bring back to the home interests and achievements which will enrich their relationship with mother herself. But if she is hostile to their friendships and sports and games, they will resent this narrowing of their lives, and their love for her will become but a cover for distrust and hatred. On the other hand, friendly contacts between the home and the school, the mother and the teacher, help both mother and children. They serve to widen the mother's understanding of the children's needs, and aid the children to feel that she is sympathetic to their wider interests and to their finding new father figures in their school world.

In what has been said so far, we have in mind mostly the ordinary family, where there has been an ordinarily good relation between the parents, with genuine goodwill, even when tempers were tried by the ups and downs of life, and occasional crises of emotion or adverse circumstance were lived through. The effect of the father's death varys with different circumstances—if, for instance, the parents have been constantly unhappy and quarrelling, if they were separated or divorced, or wanting to be so, if the father was not affectionate but hostile or quite indifferent to his children. We have no space to go into such special circumstances, however. *Sometimes* it may be an advantage to the child if the father should die; but this is seldom so. Unless his faults of character and temper are very grave, it is better for the children to have their own father throughout their years of immaturity, just as it is better if the parents can "rub along" together, even if they are far from being ideally happy.

Nor have we the space to consider in detail the differences in the child's situation according to his age when the father dies. We have pointed out that the loss of the father affects the youngest children more seriously and lastingly than it does the older members of the family.

THE FATHERLESS CHILD AT SCHOOL

To turn now to the help to fatherless children afforded by the school and social life outside the home: this is not so much a matter of special methods of education or special things to be done, as of the *attitudes* of the grown-ups, teachers and leaders. The indirect help which the school can give is more important than any explicit action.

In essence the educational needs of fatherless children are the same as those of children in ordinary circumstances, but bereaved children will be much more dependent upon a favourable atmosphere and opportunities than children who have their fathers. Their teachers have to be able to take over the authority and the guiding function of the father more adequately than with children who have actual fathers, and to give more generous interest and understanding. And this applies to girls as well as boys. It is undoubtedly desirable that fatherless girls should go to a school where some of the teachers are men.

As with the mother in the home, moreover, the teachers in the school need to recognize the depth and strength of the child's feelings as the true cause of any temporary difficulties which may appear in his work, or in his attitude to authority and to his fellows. If the importance of the death of the father is ignored or denied we are not likely to be able to help him get over such difficulties. Only if we realize their true source can we decide whether to follow a waiting policy, giving the child time to make his own inner adjustments in a friendly atmosphere, or to take some definite course of action to meet his special needs. We have first to observe and understand how far and in what way he is going to work out his own problem, how far be defeated by it.

In time of war the child is sure to have companions who are going through the same experience. Companionship in adversity is always a help, and the fact that others of his school fellows will also have lost their fathers will help the child to feel less singled out by misfortune and less guilty for the unhappy event. The older boys and girls will gain also much indirect support from discussions about the causes and course of the war, the great aims in the service of which their fathers have died. It relieves the bitterness of their loss and their envy of those who still have their fathers if these personal distresses can be related to great social purposes, the saving of past and present good and the reconstruction of the future.

One of the chief forms of help which the school can give to bereaved children is the opportunity to express their feelings in art—in painting, drawing, modelling, music, poetry and prose, the making of plays and the appreciation of drama. Very often they can express their feelings quite openly and directly in these media, and this brings great relief to inner conflict. In one Infant School in a slum area of London, years before the war, the Head Mistress was distressed because she found that the children of four years, when given plasticene for the first time, all modelled coffins, and kept on doing this for days on end! Her first impulse was to forbid this, as it horrified her so much, but having a good understanding of little children she waited and watched, and found that after a time they left this subject behind and went on to less distressing things. On talking with some of the mothers of the children who had modelled the coffins—they mostly came from one particular street near the school—she found that there had happened to be a series of deaths and funerals in this street of people whom the children knew and whose coffins they had seen. These deaths had been the centre of talk and of feeling amongst the inhabitants of the street for some weeks. The children's modelling of the coffins, in some cases with the dead person inside, was their way of externalizing the distressing and frightening images which these events had called up in their minds—of externalizing these images and mastering the feelings of unhappiness and anxiety aroused by the events. If the activity had been forbidden the children would have had to bottle up their feelings and phantasies and their emotional development would have suffered from their being deprived of a natural and healthy outlet.

The expression in various forms of art of the feelings and images aroused by the severe experience of the father's death is a most valuable aid to mental balance. It allows the child to share his experience and his inner world with others. It gives him the reassurance that something valuable can come out of the chaos of feeling, an earnest that life can triumph over death, and a proof that the grown-ups will allow him to reach out to new life in spite of father's death. Constructive handwork of all kinds has the same reassuring influence.

It can be said that, valuable as such activities—constructive handwork, creation and enjoyment in art and literature and drama—are to all children, they are quite essential for the fatherless child if he is to maintain or recover his mental health.

The opportunity for active experience in sport and games and bodily achievement of various sorts is also most helpful. Games and sports afford not only pleasurable bodily activities, but also an outlet for the ambition and the normal competitiveness which so readily becomes inhibited in the fatherless child. To struggle against others and with others, to be permitted to compete in bodily skills, provides on the one hand an approved form of "showing off", rivalry and aggression, a direct expression of these powerful instinctual forces and, on the other, a reassurance that strongly aggressive wishes do not necessarily bring great harm to others. Such activities help the boy to temper his aggression by finding appropriate channels for it which may at the same time give pleasure to others and allow them to achieve as well as himself. It eases the internal terrors of a deadly struggle between himself and his brothers, and indirectly lessens the unconscious dread that his rivalry and hostility actually brought about his father's death. It breaks through the vicious circle of feeling in which aggressive wishes towards the father automatically give rise to guilt and responsibility for what has happened to him and these feelings in their turn make him feel more aggressive and defiant.

Again, boys and girls in their teens need some definite share in governing the school community, in running camps and hostels, being to some degree and in appropriate forms responsible for order and discipline and for corporate activities. By contributing in these ways to the community of their fellows and co-operating with their elders, they gain confidence in themselves and a belief in their own future as responsible adults.

In general, friendship with older companions of both sexes, the sharing of pursuits (making useful or beautiful things, acting and singing, taking part in games and contests, country walks and interests, talk and debate) provide further outlets for feeling and a further support to the child in dealing with his sense of loss and his anxieties. Such friendly activities with friends of the same sex also make a constructive and expansive use of hidden feelings of love for them, feelings which otherwise may distort sexual development. Moreover, the giving and returning of affection between friends of both sexes allays feelings of unworthiness and guilt, and reassures the children against their phantasies of complete destruction and chaos inside. And friendships with older boys may in part take the place of the exchange of affection with a father. On the other hand, friendship with younger children often helps the older boy to feel that he in turn can be a father to younger children, recovering the lost father in himself. It helps the girl to feel that in spite of her father's death she may be able to have children of her own and to feel herself a mother towards them, thus implying that the father will be rediscovered in a future lover and husband.

Scientific studies, too, may be valuable. These in any case tend to lessen the anxieties of the ordinary boy and girl in the teens, arising from their normal sexual development. We know that adolescence is a time of great conflict, when both boy and girl struggle with the fears and doubt arising from their bodily development and the uprush of the instinctual life, together with the complex feelings of love and hate, of rivalry, hope and ambition, and the responsibilities which sexual maturing inevitably entails. Such anxieties become still more acute in fatherless children. Biological knowledge always has a steadying effect, although there will certainly be children who want to turn away altogether from biology as coming too close to personal anxieties and prefer to deal with the impersonal world of physical and mathematical science.

Even more than with children in normal circumstances, those who have lost their fathers need a wide opportunity of choice in their vocational and recreational interests and pursuits. It is impossible to say which hobby, which sort of reading and recreation, which line of work, which career, will bring most support to particular children. Their choice will depend both upon the earlier development of their inner lives and upon their personal relationship to the people they meet in these various fields of interest. What we do know is that these children need the opportunity for varied activities and rich experience; and, as far as circumstances allow, for freedom of choice.

Fatherless boys and girls at the time of adolescence, moreover, will find it helpful if they are allowed to take part in the real life of the community, outside the home and the school. We know that the majority of children suffer from the fact that they have to do this far too early, leaving school and becoming wage earners at fourteen or fifteen. But to recognize the unwisdom of ending school life and turning children into shop or factory workers so early does not mean that we should deprive boys and girls in their teens of a real place in the world, nor allow them to contribute to it in any way. There are many forms of useful social activity which they can enter into in the actual life of their neighbourhood, town or village. Examples in time of war which spring to the mind are growing vegetables in allotments and paper salvage; but such opportunities abound in time of peace as well. Growing boys and girls want and need to feel themselves useful to the community in real ways, *now*, not only in learning and when they grow up.

This proof of personal value is helpful to all but it is needed even more by children who are struggling to accept the father's death and to overcome the self-distrust it stirs up in them. And those in European lands now, whose homes have been ravaged and destroyed, could have no greater help in their own problems than being allowed to take some real and active share in the tremendous tasks which face their elders. The opportunity to give real help and have real responsibility of some sort and some degree is particularly necessary for these children in devastated countries and just as urgent as to have the chance of continuing their learning and training. To do the latter without the former would make them feel mere useless burdens and thus encourage anti-social tendencies.

In conclusion, it may be said again that some sort of emotional disturbance is very likely to arise in fatherless children. No one can predict when and how it may show itself. It may appear in any one of a variety of difficulties of behaviour and of social attitude, or in serious mental illness. On the surface there may not seem to us to be any link between the children's troublesome ways and the father's death, since the difficulties may appear some time after the event and not in obvious relation to it. But it is wise to assume that such a major event could not be without influence upon the child's development. We should always be prepared to find its effects in his emotional life and his behaviour and to allow for this in our dealings with him.

But, much as we might wish to find it, there is, we must repeat, no specific, no simple nostrum to be recommended as such, for the troubles of fatherless children. What they require in general is secure affection and friendship, understanding, patient control and guidance, positive opportunities for active and creative work and play. They need time and opportunity to mourn as well.

XIII

CHILDREN IN INSTITUTIONS[1]

(1945)

INTRODUCTORY

THE question of what measures should be taken to ensure that children who are deprived of parents and a normal home life are brought up under conditions best calculated to compensate them for the lack of parental care requires, besides a survey of the direct evidence, some consideration also of what actually constitutes good parental care, and what is the significance of the home and its usual setting in the ordinary child's life.[2]

Neither of these important questions, however, can be satisfactorily dealt with on the basis of the local experience of any single person or group of persons. For thorough understanding and wise practical decisions, it is necessary to undertake a wide survey of general experience in educational work with young children, and also a comprehensive study of development by reliable methods of scientific research.

INSTITUTIONS OR FOSTER HOMES

The first large question to be considered is whether the needs of homeless children are in general best provided for in institutions or in foster homes; and secondly, what specific conditions are required in either, if children are to thrive there—*what sort* of institution or foster home it must be.

The answer to these questions is not (at this date) a matter of mere opinion; our conclusions are reliable only if they are based upon ascertained and recorded facts.

The view is widely held among those who have studied the question that (*a*) life in an institution is *as such* definitely unfavourable to children's development, and that, other things being equal, foster homes have turned out to be more helpful; (*b*) that

---

[1] Being a Memorandum presented to the Home Office Care of Children Committee, 1945. Not previously published as a whole.
[2] I shall not be considering the large field of purely administrative questions.

certain specific psychological requirements have to be met in either case. (These will be detailed later.) A good institution may be much better than a bad foster home, and a first-rate institution better than an indifferent foster home.

The matter can be summed up by saying that whether the substitute offered to the child for a home of his own is going to be helpful or not depends entirely on how far it approximates to family life in an ordinary good home. It must be a *home*, whatever we call it, and whether it be large or small. But it is much easier for the well-chosen and supervised foster home to provide a true family life than it is for the large institution to do so.

FAMILY TIES

Social workers and students are now familiar with the vast importance of family ties in the feelings of children and ordinary parents.

E.g. in the Cambridge Evacuation Survey[1]. A report of this was published by Methuen, 1941, a study was made by various methods of investigation of the feelings of parents and children about their separation in the war, and of the reasons why children returned home against the wishes of the authorities. In many different ways the facts revealed the great strength of family ties, even in families whose homes were poor and general conditions of life were unsatisfactory. The great majority of the children felt the separation from their parents acutely, and many of their difficulties under evacuation arose from the disturbance of family relationships and the shock of separation from their parents.

This fits in with what many people have also reported when working amongst children who remained in London through the severest periods of bombing.

The view that separation from the parents and the break-up of the family seem to be far more adverse to children's development and mental health than the physical threat of danger and death is widely held among psychologists and social workers generally.

EXAMPLES OF DIRECT EVIDENCE

Let us now consider some samples of the evidence for the view

[1] *The Cambridge Evacuation Survey*, Methuen & Co., 1941. Edited by Susan Isaacs, S. Clement Brown and R. H. Thouless.

that institution life is *as such* unfavourable to the child's development. It must be remembered that there will always be exceptions to the general rule. Institutions vary; and in any case, every institution can (fortunately) show its examples of children who have done well. We have, however, to consider *general tendencies*, and the effect on the *majority* of the inmates.

(1) In a recent authoritative survey of scientific studies of the development of personality throughout childhood[1] the authors touch upon the problem of homeless children as follows: " . . . it is commonly believed by experienced social workers that supervised foster home placements of dependent children are far preferable to institutional placements from the standpoint of both physical and emotional health. Naturally, in an individual case, a choice would be determined by the particular institutions and foster homes available . . .

"Theis, for example, reported upon two groups of foster children, who had been placed (in foster homes) after the age of five. The 111 children of one group had spent at least five years in orphan asylums before placement; 34 per cent. proved to be in adult life 'incapable'. Among these incapables were 13.5 per cent. classified as 'harmful' or 'on trial'. In the other group, numbering ninety-seven, none had lived in orphanages; only 18 per cent. were incapable, and only 6 per cent. delinquent or 'on trial'. The author states that there was no difference in family backgrounds of the two groups, and little difference in age at placement, but does not give precise data upon these points."

(2) "The unfavourable influence[2] of the institutional environment is noticeable even in the earliest period of life. Gindl and Hetzer tested 60 children, 20 institution, 20 foster, and 20 very much neglected family children, all between 1 and 12 years of age, using the Hetzer-Koller (30) test series for the 2nd year. Table 9 (below) presents these results. In spite of the good health condition of the institution children, they were mentally more retarded than neglected family children, not to speak of the foster children. This last result has been confirmed in an investigation with 275 Austrian foster families." (Danziger, Hetzer, Löw-Beer.)

---

[1] *Personality Development in Childhood*, by Mary Cover Jones and Barbara Stoddard Burks, Monographs of the Society for Research in Child Development, Vol. I, No. 4 Washington, D.C., 1936.
[2] "The Social Behaviour of the Child," Charlotte Bühler, Chapter 12 of *Handbook of Child Psychology*, edited by Carl Murchison, 1931, Oxford University Press, p. 421.

Environmental Situation.		Hetzer-Koller Development Test.	Hetzer-Reindorf Language Test.
Children from institutions	.. ..	47	36
Neglected family children	.. ..	78	80
Foster children	.. ..	90	95

(3) "The hospitalised infant[1] sleeps less, passes more stools, is more liable to respiratory infection, than the infant at home. Also there is a dulling of response to emotional stimuli—e.g. these infants do not smile in response to mother at three months of age. There is a lowering of resistance and delay or distortion in development.

"When a child's mother is excluded from hospital, with a high level of bodily hygiene, mortality is high. When children were mothered by nurses and doctors, and parents' visits were allowed, mortality fell sharply.

"This applied also to toddlers. E.g. there was a hospital case in which a young child went steadily downhill until 'so weak that it seemed he might stop breathing at any minute'. The child then returned to the mother—rapid and complete recovery followed."

(4) "Pediatricians[2] have long recognized that the failure of infants to thrive in institutions is dependent, for the most part, on lack of the kind of stimulation which they normally receive at home from the mother. Infants in hospitals are lonely. In an attempt to compensate for the deficiencies of hospitals in this respect, at Bellevue Hospital nurses and interns are encouraged to handle the infants at every opportunity and parents are invited to visit their infants. That these measures have not adversely affected the health of infants is shown by the marked drop in the infant case fatality rate in the children's medical service of Bellevue Hospital during the past ten years." (From Author's Summary; quoted in *Child Development Abstracts*.)

(5) "The book[3] stresses the importance of mothering in the emotional life of the infant as being 'as vital to the child's development as food'. By expressing consistent tender, caressing love, the mother teaches the small baby to love, and this has far-reaching effects on later life, for 'the capacity for mature emotional relationships in adult life is a direct outgrowth of the mothering which an infant receives'. There is need to stress this

---

[1] "Loneliness in Infancy," Bakwin, *American Journal Diseases of Children*, 1942.
[2] "Loneliness in Infants," Dr. Harry Bakwin. *American Journal of Diseases of Children*. 63: 30–40.
[3] *The Rights of Infants: Early Psychological Needs and their Satisfaction*, Margaret A. Ribble. Columbia University Press: New York, 1943.

phase of child care. There are advocates of institutional or group care for young children; many professional workers with children and many mothers do not appreciate the importance of the emotional attachment of mother and baby". (Quotation from *Child Development Abstracts*.)

(6) Dr. Marjorie MacRae has reported to me verbally that she had noticed striking changes in children from London institutions who had been evacuated during the war to foster homes in the Hertfordshire area; how they gradually became "much more human", more natural in the expression of their feelings, more lively, more trusting, more outgoing. She attributed this to the fact that they were now in ordinary homes with a natural relationship to ordinary human surroundings and foster parents, as compared with the rigid routine and emotionally barren life of an institution.

(7) "The Brown personality inventory[1] was given to groups of institutionalized children (200 orphans), to groups of several hundred children living with their parents in the general population, and to a group of children in the general population whose parents were of low socio-economic status (100 boys). It was found that the neuroticism of institution children (mean score, boys = 23.93; girls = 29.07) was greater than that of children who lived with their parents in the general population (mean score, boys = 17.34; girls = 18.36) while there was a similarity between them and the other group of low socio-economic status (mean score = 22.75)." (Quotation from *Child Development Abstracts*.)

(8) "This[2] is a report of one phase of an experimental, observational and case history investigation of fifteen adolescents whose rearing in the first three years of life had been in an infant institution and whose subsequent experience was in foster homes (institution group). These children were contrasted with an equated group of fifteen children whose major life experience had been with foster families and whose total experience had been with families (foster home group). The institution children show a greater trend to deviation from the 'normal' Graphic Rorschach pattern than do the foster home children. This deviation manifests itself in an unusual adherence to the 'concrete' attitude and in

[1] "Neuroticism of Institution Versus Non-Institution Children," Fred Brown, *Journal of Applied Psychology*, 21: 379–383, 1937.
[2] "The Effects of Early Institutional Care on Adolescent Personality (Graphic Rorschach Data)," William Goldfarb, *Child Development*, 14: 213–223, 1943.

inadequate conceptualization. Finally this 'concretivity' is specifically represented in such qualities as apathy in relation to environment and behaviour that is unreflective, unaccountable and without conscious purpose. Thus the Graphic Rorschach data tend to confirm the findings and conclusions based on other investigative devices. These also show the institution child to be clearly differentiated from the foster home child. The following essential traits in the institution child are inferred from the mass of data: (1) an impoverished, undifferentiated personality with deficiency in inhibition and control, and (2) passivity or apathy of personality." (Quotation from *Child Development Abstracts*.)

(9) "The subjects of this study[1] were two groups of forty foster children each. One group included children who had been in an institution from early infancy to about age three years; the other, children who had been in foster homes from early infancy. The two groups were equated within three months on the basis of both age and length of time under care, with the minimum chronological age set at six years. Two check lists of problem behaviour were employed. Both groups demonstrated all the different kinds of problem behavior noted in the lists, though to a differing degree. Except for withdrawal behavior and anxieties related to intra-family relationships (in which foster home children tended to exceed the institution children) the foster home children tended to show less of the various kinds of problem behavior. The institution children seemed to be more frequently characterized by the need for adult attention, problems of restlessness, hyper-activity, inability to concentrate, restlessness in sleep, craving for affection, sensitivity, attention-getting behavior, selfishness in play and lack of popularity with other children, disobedience, temper display, and stealing." (Quotation from *Child Development Abstracts*.)

(10) "The adjustment of older children[2] who have spent several years in an institution to community living involves certain special difficulties," says Miss Verry, executive secretary of the Chicago Orphan Asylum. "First, there is the problem of economic adjustment—of getting and spending money; second, the problem of living with relatives in a family group; third, the

---

[1] "Infant Rearing and Problem Behaviour," William Goldfarb, *American Journal of Orthopsychiatry*, 13: 249–265.
[2] "Problems Facing Children Who Have Had a Relatively Long Period of Institutional Care," Ethel Verry, *Child Welfare League of America Bulletin*, 18, No. 2: 2–3, 6–7, 1939.

problem of making friends and creating a satisfying social and recreational life; and fourth, the problem of marriage and parenthood. The over-protection of children, a danger in institutional care," Miss Verry points out, "increases the difficulty of the adjustments to ordinary living that the child must make." (Quotation from *Child Development Abstracts*.)

(11) Here is an account[1] of the results of caring for children in a specially favourable small "home", where psychological and educational (as well as medical) skill of a high order was drawn upon to create a good family atmosphere:

"A new class of institutional child has come into being during the past ten years or so: this is the baby reared in the 'home management house' of a college or university. Vance, Prall, Simpson, and McLaughlin have reported upon thirteen such infants (of ages five to seventeen months), comparing their development with small control groups. The 'home management' children, as a group, excelled the groups in boarding homes and in an orphanage in every aspect of behavior studies—intellectual, motor, and language development, adaptive behavior and personal-social behavior as appraised by the Gesell schedule."

These quotations from the scientific literature of child development may suffice to indicate how widely held and how well substantiated by direct evidence is the view that formal institutional life, or any situation in which intimate personal contacts of a family type are excluded, is definitely unfavourable to healthy development of mind and body.

Among the adverse results which *tend* to occur and which have been reliably recorded in a large number of cases are: Retardation of physical growth and greater proneness to ill-health (especially in infants and young children); retardation of mental growth (in language and in manipulative skill); lack of adaptability, of reflectiveness, or self-control, impoverishment of personality, apathy, aloofness, rigidity of social response, lack of social feeling; greater frequency of anti-social behaviour and delinquency; greater tendency to neurosis. Or again in other cases problems of behaviour, such as restlessness, hyper-activity, inability to concentrate, restlessness in sleep, craving for affection, sensitivity, attention-getting behaviour, selfishness in play and

[1] *Personality Development in Childhood*, Mary Cover Jones and Barbara Stoddard Burks, Monographs of the Society for Research in Child Development, Vol. I, No. 4, Washington, D.C., 1936.

lack of popularity with other children, disobedience, temper display, and stealing; difficulties in finding friends or dealing with money, etc. (in adolescence).

All these characteristics which institution children tend to show are more strongly marked in the case of the children who enter institutions at an early age.

It may be repeated that no one suggests that these undesirable results are found with every child or in every institution; but that, on the comparative data, *a strong tendency is noted for children in institutions to show such difficulties more frequently and to a greater degree than children in their own homes or in foster homes.*

WHY ARE INSTITUTIONS UNFAVOURABLE?

What characteristics of life in institutions are responsible for these tendencies to various sorts of adverse development in their inmates? This involves a reference to normal children and normal conditions.

Evidence as to the general question of what are favourable and unfavourable conditions for normal development may be drawn from two main sorts of observation and research: (1) the study of well-adjusted normal children in various circumstances and classes of society; (2) the study of those children (and adults) whose development has gone wrong, who have become neurotic or delinquent, or show special difficulties of behaviour. By bringing these two sets of facts together we are able to arrive at some conclusion as to the most essential needs of young children.

ESSENTIAL NEEDS OF CHILDREN

I shall now summarise briefly my views as to the most essential needs of young children, those which must be met if their development is to be normal, again quoting evidence or opinions from other authors at various points. I shall select only those aspects which bear closely upon the subject of this enquiry.

What I have to say will mostly refer to the infant and the very young child, since on the one hand it is the early years which are the most formative, and on the other, it is in these years that the social and emotional needs of the child are most readily overlooked. The infant and young child are so often unable to make their troubles known, whereas the older child and adolescent reveal them not only through speech but also through defiant or delinquent behaviour, through running away and other forms of protest. But it is the conditions of life in the earliest years which will most fully determine the future—whether the child becomes mentally ill or delinquent, or develops into a useful citizen and a satisfactory parent.

The essential needs of children can be grouped under the two headings: (A) Human Relationships; and (B) Activities.

A. *Human Relationships*

Essential needs under this heading can be summarised as:

1. Affection.
2. Security.
3. Mild control.
4. Companionship with other children.

The following considerations have to be borne in mind:

(*a*) Throughout early childhood the world is a *personal* world, for the child's mind. Everything is for him centred in persons. All that happens is attributed to the will of human beings; there are no neutral impersonal events. The infant's wishes and aims are focused upon his mother. He is at first entirely dependent upon her for his existence and his satisfactions, and his mind is built upon this pattern. The whole structure of the young child's being is orientated to personal relationships—first of all to his mother, and later to his father and other adults as well.

Professor Jean Piaget,[1] of the University of Geneva, has studied many fundamental aspects of the intellectual growth and social development of children, from birth to adolescence, by means of observations and experiments on large numbers of children.

Among the points from his researches, supported by a wealth of evidence and relevant to this enquiry, is his conclusion that the world of the infant and young child is always a *personal* world. Neutral things and impersonal happenings come into the child's awareness only slowly and relatively late. His observations, his thoughts and his feelings tend to be centred in persons—and in his early years, in his parents. This is shown in many detailed ways: e.g., in the very young child's mind every object is alive, even sticks and stones. These things can feel and have purpose. Later on he believes that everything that moves is alive (even the wind, the sun and the moon). Later still he distinguishes between

[1] His conclusions have been published in a series of important books translated into English, and published by Kegan Paul: *The Language and Thought of the Child; The Child's Conception of the World; Judgement and Reasoning in the Child; The Child's Conception of Causality; The Moral Judgement of the Child;* and others.

things that are alive because they can feel as well as move (animals and human beings) and inanimate objects, which do not move of their own accord and do not feel.

Moreover, everything in the world (even things like mountains and lakes and rivers) has been made either by men (fathers) or by God for the purposes of men. Every event in the world (including the movement of sun and stars, the blowing of the wind, etc.), happens through forces or purposes inherent in objects; and ultimately these purposes are *moral* ones. The very young child has little notion of merely physical causality. Causal relationships are to him mainly moral and personal. Things happen in order "to keep people good" or "to punish them because they are bad".

Moreover the morality of the very small child is an intensely severe and strict one. Piaget's evidence confirms what has often been observed in the spontaneous dramatic play of little children, that the young child feels his parents to be *either* ideally good *or* terribly severe, inflicting lethal punishments. All that happens is thus (in the child's mind) the outcome of the goodness or badness, the lovingness or cruelty, of his parents (or the parent-substitutes in charge of him)—and of his own feelings and behaviour towards them.

(*b*) In the infant and young child, feelings are very intense and overwhelming, and imagination is very vivid. The child's behaviour and his picture of the external world are more determined, in the early years, by his inner world of feeling and imagination than by what is real from the adult point of view. What people do to him and around him is necessarily interpreted in terms of his own feelings. This makes the behaviour of the grown-ups not less, but *more* important. The child is even more dependent upon the goodness or badness of the adults around him that he would be if he had an adult sense of reality. What from the adult point of view is a mild deprivation or small discomfort or punishment may be felt by the child to be overwhelmingly severe.

(*c*) In the young child's mind, moreover, people are *always* either good or bad. Mere indifference on their part is felt by him to be a positive badness. If they satisfy his needs by loving and caring for him, they are felt to be "good" parents. And not only if they tantalise or hurt him, but if they neglect him or leave him without guidance and control, they are felt to be "bad". And in the very young child, these patterns of "good" and "bad" are extreme in character. Mother is (at first) felt to be either *wholly* loving and helpful, or wholly hostile and cruel. If she is cold and neglectful, then he feels starved and helpless, and everything becomes bad to him. In the same way, if he is living in an institution, and finds nobody to give him warm human contact because people are either indifferent or too busy, this does not mean to him the mere *absence* of the good he requires, a merely neutral place; it means the actual presence of positive evil. The people around him are felt to be actively unfriendly and cruel; they starve his feelings even if they feed his body. Conditions which from the point of view of the adult may seem satisfactory because the child is well fed and housed, kept clean and given schooling, may to him be entirely barren and hostile because his *emotional* needs are not met.

In other words, the world as it appears to the young child's mind is very like that of the old fairy tales. When he feels loved and satisfied, the world seems full of fairy godmothers and helpful genii, bringing good things by beneficent magic; when he feels neglected and unloved, the world seems full of witches and ogres, terrible giants, bad fairies, who deprive and destroy by an evil magic.

Moreover, what he will become as an adult citizen is determined quite as much by his feelings and his imaginative apprehension of the people around him as it is by his being fed and medically cared for, or given good schooling in later childhood. It has been established, for example, that delinquent children at any age are still living (in their inner beliefs) in the world of giants and ogres. Their anti-social conduct is partly the result of their hidden (largely unconscious) terror of cruel tyrants and extremely severe punishments, which yet paradoxically they feel compelled to defy. Or they may be led to provoke punishment in order to exchange their awful phantasies for a less unbearable reality.

Only as the sense of reality slowly develops (in normal children) through the early years, fostered by the real experience of affection, security and mild control from his parents or those who stand for parents, does the child's inner world of feeling come closer to the actual human world of ordinary people who are neither fairy godmothers nor evil giants; a world of social realities in which the child can take his own place.

(*d*) Children become adapted to this real world, become social beings themselves, able to exercise a self-control and to co-operate with others in an active and friendly but responsible way, *not* by virtue of what they are taught in words, but by living experience of people, by absorbing the pattern of behaviour shown in the actual personalities of those around them. The child cannot judge father and mother and teacher except by their behaviour and their emotional attitudes towards him. Words, verbal commandments, abstract principles, have no significance except in so far as they are embodied in the actions and the personalities of the people upon whom he is dependent. What parents and teachers are, and his real experience of them, is infinitely more important than what they profess or claim to be, or tell him he ought to be. This fact is no new discovery—"Example is better than precept" is a well-known truth. But the experience of the psychologist has confirmed and amplified this truth in a new way by his understanding of the deeper, more hidden processes in the child's mind. Put concretely, it is useless to tell the child to be kind and loving and self-controlled, considerate with others, etc., if he does not experience these virtues in the day-to-day conduct and attitudes of the adults about him towards him and towards other children. If he is in fact treated coldly and distantly or harshly, starved of affection and natural human contacts, he cannot himself become a social being, trustful of other people and confident in his own ability to be decent and generous.

(*e*) His first essential need is thus *affection*, the experience of loving care, either from his own actual parents or from those who take over the function of parents, whether in a foster home or an institution. The experience of love is just as necessary for the child's mental and moral growth as good food and medical care are necessary for his bodily health and development. Even his bodily health is greatly influenced (especially in infancy and early childhood) by the happiness or unhappiness which comes from experiencing love, or the lack of it—as the evidence quoted above from Dr. Bakwin's records shows.

The evidence as to the absolute need of the infant and young child for love from his parents, expressed in all the stuff of day to day experience (being talked to and played with, as well as fed and clothed) is unchallengeable.

E.g. (1) Dr. Florence Powdermaker, a psychiatrist in New

York, gave me the following evidence verbally some years ago.

In a Home for the care and treatment of adolescent delinquent girls, records were kept for several years of the response to treatment of each of the girls and of her later history after she was discharged from the Home. (The Home provided skilled medical care, individual psychiatric treatment, and training in various occupations, with preparation for social life.) After a number of years, the records were analysed by outside people in order to measure the success or failure of the treatment given as indicated by the later history of the girls. It was found that the treatment had been successful in 50 per cent. of the cases. Half of the girls had remained free of delinquent behaviour and were well adapted to social life.

Of the 50 per cent. failures, those who did not respond to the care and treatment provided in the Home, but returned to criminal ways after their discharge, a detailed study was made of their earliest history. It was found in every one of these cases that the girls had suffered severely from lack of affection in the first two years of life. The circumstances varied: some had lost both parents, some were illegitimate and badly treated, some had bad parents, cruel or anti-social. The common element amongst these varied histories was the lack of love and security which they experienced during the first two years of life.

(2) Here is an account of a useful experiment in different ways of treating orphan children within the same institution.[1]

"Amy Daniels directed by Bird Baldwin, in an experimental child study of this development phase (i.e. two years) was able to show the far-reaching importance of sympathetic individual care. Two groups of two-year-old children living in the same institution were segregated from each other and subjected to two divergent types of treatment. One group was given very little tenderness although adequately cared for in every other respect. In the other group, a nurse was assigned to each child and there was no lack of tenderness and affection. At the end of half a year the first group was mentally and physically retarded, in comparison with the second. In order to effect normal psychic and physical maturity, individual care and devotion are indispensable in the upbringing of small children."

"It is clear that the child needs individual care, particularly at this stage of its development. The removal therefore of children

[1] From Birth to Maturity, Charlotte Bühler, Kegan Paul, 1935, p. 65.

from their homes to institutions is more harmful at this age (two years) than at any other."

(3) Further evidence is offered by Dr. John Bowlby's investigation into the history and psychology of juvenile thieves.[1]

Dr. Bowlby investigated the characters and home life of forty-four juvenile thieves referred to a Child Guidance Clinic. Their histories and psychological characteristics were closely compared with the same number of non-delinquent children, a "Control Group", also referred to the Clinic but for other troubles. Among his conclusions the following points are relevant to this enquiry:

"The thieves are classified according to their characters. Only 2 were regarded as fairly 'Normal' emotionally, 9 were Depressed, 2 Circular, 13 Hyperthymic, 14 of a character type which has been christened 'Affectionless' and 4 Schizoid or Schizophrenic. There are no Affectionless Characters amongst the controls, a difference which is significant" (p. 126).

"Seventeen of the thieves had suffered complete and prolonged separation (six months or more) from their mothers or established foster-mothers during their first five years of life. Only two controls had suffered similar separations, a statistically significant difference. Twelve of the 14 thieves who were of the Affectionless Character had suffered a prolonged separation in contrast to only 5 of the remaining 30 thieves, a difference which is again significant. Clinical evidence is presented which shows that a prolonged separation is a principal cause of the Affectionless (and delinquent) Character" (p. 127).

"The relationship of stealing to truancy and sexual offences is discussed. Evidence is advanced that the Affectionless Character is prone to both, and that a substantial proportion of prostitutes are probably of this character" (p. 127).

". . . if early diagnosis is important, how much more vital is prevention. Certain factors, it is true, cannot be prevented. Deaths, whether of mother or little brother, will occur, but even here an understanding of the child's emotions may enable timely help to be given. Anxious and nagging mothers also may always be with us, but again an understanding of their problem and the provision of play centres and nursery schools will go far to ameliorate the lot of their children. . . The prolonged separation of young children from their mothers may also on occasion

---

[1] "Forty-four Juvenile Thieves: Their Characters and Home-Life," *International Journal of Psycho-Analysis*, Vol. XXV, Pts. I and II, 1944, and Pts. III and IV, 1944.

be unavoidable. Nevertheless, if all those who had to advise on the upbringing of small children, and not least among them doctors, were aware of the appalling damage which separations of this kind have on the development of a child's character, many could be avoided and many of the most distressing cases of chronic delinquency prevented" (p. 126).

Dr. Bowlby's evidence thus brings out the far-reaching effects of early and prolonged separations from the mother, a conclusion which fits in with the other evidence in favour of the view that personal relationships, particularly with the parents, are of the utmost importance for the child's development, and that if circumstances of one sort or another deprive the children of this relationship with their own parents it is essential that satisfactory parent-substitutes and foster homes should be provided.

(*f*) Another essential need of the infant and young child is *security*. He needs to feel safe in his environment, safe not only from physical dangers and discomforts, but also from shocks in his personal life, such as frequent and unexpected changes in the people upon whom he is dependent, and to whom he has become attached. He needs not only a regular routine in his daily life, a rhythm of bodily care suited to his age, but also a stable relationship with people. If his nurse is frequently changed, as may happen in an institution (or in comfortable families which employ nursemaids), this shocks his feelings in a way which is very hard to bear, and makes it difficult for him to build up stable attitudes of affection, of trust in others and confidence in his own feelings. Many children who have this experience tend to withdraw from affectionate relationships altogether, becoming suspicious, distrustful and aloof, since they never know what to expect. What is the good of loving if one so often loses the object of one's love and has constantly to make a fresh start? In the ordinary home this sort of thing does not often happen; but there is sometimes an insecurity arising from changeable moods in mother or father. The mother who indulges one day and scolds the next is a great trial to the child and arouses similar feelings of insecurity and uncertainty. The "spoilt" child is an anxious child. He is "spoilt" not by too much loving but by fickle indulgence and a mixture of uneasy and changeable feelings in his mother. A steady emotional attitude and consistent ways of teaching and training are a very necessary support to the child.

This unfulfilled need of the child for a stable relationship with one person or a small group of persons who remain in constant touch with him, whom he can dare to love and upon whom he can depend, is one of the most serious lacks in institutional life, orphanages or nursery homes for infants and young children. It may be difficult to avoid, but must be faced and overcome. Whatever the practical difficulties of organisation, homes and institutions for young children must safeguard their emotional development, since the future social development of the child— whether he becomes ill, delinquent or a useful citizen, depends more upon this than upon any other factor. If he learns to be distrustful and aloof when he is young, he will never become a well adjusted person in later life, able to get on with his family, friends and employers, and to meet the demands of the community with confidence.

(g) The great help which consistent methods of handling and training the child bring to his development links with another essential need, the need for a steady but mild *control*. This is another aspect of good parenthood. The good parent not only gives love to the child but helps him to control his own aggression and destructive impulses. The small child *is* aggressive; he is greedy to get all he wants, he is full of rivalry and jealousy towards other children and grown-ups, he gets angry and often feels great rages if he cannot get what he wishes for, and even in cooler moments he may hate other children or may damage physical objects or destroy things he values. He is at the same time very frightened about these aggressive impulses. He becomes very anxious if he believes that the grown-ups cannot control him, because he feels he cannot control himself. Self-control does develop later (although even the adolescent boy or girl suffers acute anxiety about his wishes and impulses and the feeling that he cannot yet control the uprush of his instinctual life which new bodily development is now bringing). The young child feels even more the need of some controlling influence. That there should be such an influence is a familiar fact, which is in no danger of being overlooked in institutions, or in most foster-homes. We all know that it is chiefly fond mothers who are over-indulgent with their own children. What is not always realised, however, is that if the control which the child seeks, as a help in keeping himself in order and saving the persons and objects he loves from his destructive impulses, is to be really educative and help him to become an independent, self-controlled citizen, it must be a *mild* and loving control. Severe punishments are quite as unwise and unfruitful as indulgence and the lack of control. Mild control by a firm and just authority is always felt by the child to be a help. This educates him in self-control. Harsh punishments, rigid prohibitions of natural pleasures and healthy activities serve to increase the child's hate, aggression and anxiety, and are far more likely to turn him into a delinquent than into a useful member of society.

Moreover, control should be primarily a *positive* control (as it usually is in the hands of a skilful school teacher), relying upon the provision of positive means of activity rather than upon negative prohibitions. Not so much: "You must *not* do that," as "You *may* do this, and here is the means to do it". To provide for constructive and co-operative occupations and responsibilities is the best form of control. (This point links with what we shall have to say in the next section about children's activities.)

If, then, the child's parents are so enormously important to him and his need for affection, security and a wise control is so great, how does this bear upon the needs of children whose parents are either dead or absent or so unsatisfactory that society decides to remove the children from their care? It means that whatever substitutes we make for the child's own home and own parents, these must, if they are going to help his development, come as near as possible to being good *parents*, and must be felt by the child to represent *good* parents. In the case of bad homes, it is not enough to take the child's own parents away and then supply simply the physical basis of life. To have no parents at all (as in a formal institution) is a positive evil and scarcely less undesirable for the child than having actively bad parents of his own. If the representatives of society decide to take the grave step of separating the child from his own parents, they must realise that this *is* a very grave step and that they then have the further responsibility of recreating a family life for the child. Otherwise they themselves become *bad* parents both in fact and in the child's mind. Again, if the child has no parents of his own and society takes the responsibility of putting him in a home where his bodily needs are met, this still meets only one partial aspect of his needs as a human being. To shirk or evade the responsibility for satisfying his emotional and social requirements is for society's representatives to act as bad parents themselves.

There is, however, still another essential need of the child in the world of human relationships, viz. the need for active *companionship* with other children. It is largely by means of an active sharing of work and play in a genuine social life with other children that the young child learns to overcome his distrust of himself and others and his rivalry with them, to build up a true social feeling of comradely affection and group loyalty. Here again, it must be emphasised that the transformation of the child into a social being does not come about by his being talked to and preached to, but only by active *experiences* in making and doing and sharing and playing and working with other children in day-to-day social participation.

Institution life does, of course, bring the child contact with others. Unfortunately, it tends to be mostly a limited and passive contact, governed by strict rules in which the natural interchange of talk and the natural sharing in play and constructive activity are either forbidden (through most of the day) or confined within the narrowest limits. Moreover, the number of children in a group is so often far too large. The young child cannot make contact of feeling with large numbers of other children. He is at home only in a group of about the size of an ordinary large family. His feelings of trust and confidence are overwhelmed by anxiety in too big a group, whether of his own age or of different ages. Life in most institutions thus not only baulks the child of his natural experience of active play with his fellows, but stimulates his fear and distrust of them by keeping him constantly in the presence of other children with whom he can have no active relationship.

All this bears very closely upon the size of the group of which the young child should be made a member. It is quite essential for his social development that whatever the size of the institution as such, he should feel himself to be a member of a small family group of other children, each one of which can be a real live person to him and interchange experiences and feelings with him. He needs varied contacts, but they have to be alive and real.

It is not, of course, only a matter of numbers, of the size of the group the child is in contact with, but also of the internal relationships, the form and method of control, the nature of the activities for which opportunities and material are provided. This brings us to consider the activities provided for children.

B. *Activities*

I have already pointed out the emotional need of children for social life and the fact that they cannot become responsible citizens without satisfaction of their natural longings for social contacts with their fellows. I have also emphasised that their social life needs to be an *active* one. It is not the mere presence of other children but active participation with them, doing real things together, an active interchange of feeling and experience, which educates the child.

Having the chance to develop bodily skills and to co-operate in play and in learning is of tremendous help not only to the child's physical health but also to his emotional life and mental balance. It gives him hope and confidence in his own future as a grown-up, and trust in the parents (or parent-substitutes) as people who will allow and encourage him to become grown-ups like themselves.

NATURAL ACTIVITIES OF A FAMILY HOME

This applies not only to the development of manipulative skills in creative handwork but also to participation in the daily activities of the home, helping to keep it clean and orderly. Every young child wishes to help his mother in the work of the home, especially at the nursery ages. Later on he may rebel against too much of this, especially if he is expected to do it and it takes the place of free, natural play out of doors; but within the limits of his ability, he does wish to share in the daily routine of the home, and to become independent in looking after himself.

A comparison was recently made in Chicago[1] of two groups of young children of nursery school ages: (*a*) those from homes (their own homes) where the children were allowed to help their mothers up to the limit of their ability—feeding, washing and dressing themselves, dusting, sweeping, washing crockery, etc. (Positive ideal of children's goodness.) (*b*) Children from (own) homes where they were expected to be very obedient, very quiet and mostly passive. (Negative ideal of children's goodness.) It was found that children from the first sort of homes had fewer tantrums, were less liable to be obstinate or disobedient, or to refuse a request from their parents, and had better bodily health than those from the second type of home.

Moreover, active social participation, playing with other

[1] *The Observation of Children*, by Mrs. Alschuler.

children and talking to grown-ups, such as happens naturally in the everyday life of an ordinary family, makes a great contribution to the child's intellectual life as well. It stimulates his wish to speak and his understanding of language, and by the asking and answering of questions it stirs his interest in the multifarious activities of the real world and continually adds to his knowledge and enlarges his perceptions and understanding in a pleasurable way.

In a basic study by M. Sturm (summarized by C. Bühler),[1] twenty-four hour observation of children between the ages of nine months and six years brought out significant quantitative differences between stimulating factors in homes and in institutions. "The family child has a great many more social contacts during the day than does the institution child. Such contacts as the institution child does have appear to be far less favourable for mental and personality growth. He receives more orders, asks fewer questions, and receives fewer explanations."

Again, in a valuable study[2] made some years ago by two parents of the various questions asked by their boy between three and seven years of age, it was found that by far the most active questioning, the greatest number of questions which could be called "scientific", questions as to how things were made, what they did, what they were for, how they worked, were asked in the moment-to-moment interchange of questions and answers with an interested mother and father in the two fundamental situations of ordinary life in a home: viz. (a) being bathed and cleansed, watching the water flow into and out of the bath, making a lather with the soap, and so on; (b) eating, cooking, shopping, and everything to do with food and feeding, at the meal table, and in the kitchen.

In most institutions, children suffer from a lack of the continuous stimulus which such basic events in the ordinary work of maintaining life can yield, especially when they are shared and talked about with persons who are interested in what the child thinks and feels about his experiences, and patient enough to answer his questions.

Talking with people is one aspect of the natural activities of the child which educate him. Others are (a) the chance to develop bodily skills by making use of natural interests (running, jumping,

[1] Op. cit.
[2] *The Scientific Interests of a Five Year Old Boy*, by Two Parents.

climbing, throwing, learning to play games, dancing, various forms of sport, etc.; (b) the opportunity of developing manipulative skill in various forms of making and doing, in creative handwork and art; (c) active planning and achieving in various forms of study. Learning in the 3 R's, history, geography and other school subjects, is much more effective when the children are active agents in the pursuit of knowledge, rather than passive recipients of what is taught; (d) contact with the world outside the home (whether this be the child's own home, a foster home or an institution), contact with the real world of adult life and its economic, industrial and social activities.

STIMULATING MATERIALS

The ordinary comfortable home, moreover, provides many playthings and materials for inventive play and creative activities —not only by way of the toys, tools and stuffs specially bought for the child, but also in the ordinary objects and utensils and odds and ends of material of the day-to-day household life—such as pots and pans, pebbles, matches, dough, cotton reels, paper, rags and boxes. The very poor home has much less to offer, but may still be rich in this respect as compared with the war nursery or the regulated institution. These often provide extremely little in the way of materials for the child's imaginative use and pleasurable enjoyment.

Charlotte Bühler,[1] after great experience in observing and testing the development of young children, remarks: "It is possible that a child who is given no materials to work with, may as a result be mentally retarded. This happens frequently with children who are brought up in institutions. Institutions as a rule maintain a very high standard of hygiene, but are rather backward psychologically and pedagogically. Children from well-to-do homes give the impression in the first grade of being especially bright largely in consequence of their having been provided with constructive play materials."

Again, she says:

"Let us now consider the environment of the child under discussion. It comes from an institution where there were almost no play opportunities and only very minimal contact with grown-ups. These factors alone would suffice to explain the child's

[1] Op. cit., p. 120.

low-grade social response. Why, however, is the child's response to material inadequate?

"In the test situation this child's initial response both to toys and to the examiner was one of shock. The child cried and sat motionless in front of the toys. In the course of the next two-and-a-half hours, being left alone, it gradually became accustomed to the toys and carried out some of the movements that we expect from a child of its age.[1] We find this sort of response among those children who have no opportunities to play with toys, who find neither encouragement nor stimulation in their surroundings and who require several hours in the test situation before they can overcome their psychic inertia, and respond to the stimuli that are presented."

It is essential in any environment to provide for the children's manipulative and imaginative play and their creative activities, by generous material, which need never be costly, but should be suitable for each successive age.

Active Use of Materials by Children

The last quotations will have suggested how important it is for young children to have *free use* of various materials. It is of comparatively little value for them in the earlier school years to follow a prescribed programme of formal work.

The value of active methods of learning has been fully demonstrated by a number of recent experiments and investigations.

Miss E. R. Boyce's account[2] of her very valuable work in an Infant School in a slum district of London should be considered. The school was in an ordinary school building and ordinarily equipped; the children came from the poorest sort of home, the general conditions of their lives being very unfavourable. Yet, by starting from the children's spontaneous play and giving them active methods of learning throughout their work, she enabled the children to become socially independent and co-operative, interested and alert in all their daily experiences in their ordinary lives, very responsive to the experiences they gained in the school work, and well ahead (allowing for their level of intelligence) in the 3 R's and other school occupations. The school became for the children a place where they were

[1] Op. cit., p. 35.
[2] *Play in the Infants' School*, by E. R. Boyce, Methuen, 1938.

happy and eager to learn, and *able* to learn up to the full limits of their natural ability.

Her book is a clear proof of the value of those methods which make use of the children's activities.

Another recent research which demonstrates the value of making use of the children's activities in learning is a comparison of different educational methods in the Infant and Junior School by D. E. M. Gardner (now Head of the Department of Child Development, University of London Institute of Education). Miss Gardner[1] compared two different types of Infant School, taking a number of each type which were the best of their kind: (*a*) those which relied upon the activity of the children as a means of learning, methods which utilised their natural forms of play and allowed them to move about in the classroom and do practical work, talk and play with each other; and (*b*) those in which the children sat still and quiet at their desks and were taught on routine class lines, according to formal schemes planned by the teacher.

Miss Gardner chose schools which were similar in economic status and social surroundings, and children who were of approximately the same distribution of intelligence in each type of school. She tested the various aspects of the children's development some years later, and her results were very clear. The schools using "activity methods" were superior to a greater or lesser degree in every significant test, with the exception of writing (at six years of age). I shall quote her own summary of results. (The schools described as "experimental" were the ones allowing children to be active; the "controls" were those using more formal methods of teaching.)

---

[1] *Testing Results in the Infant School,* by D. E. M. Gardner, Methuen, 1 42.

SUMMARY OF RESULTS

(a) *Tests in which the experimental schools were distinctly superior.*

1. Assembling material ingeniously to make interesting pictures.
2. Free drawing and painting and expressing imaginative ideas through drawing.
3. Answering specific questions asked, making good sentences, and expressing themselves spontaneously in words.
4. Showing a friendly and responsive attitude to a strange adult.
5. Good social behaviour towards other children.
6. Writing quickly and neatly at seven and eight years old.
7. Concentration on a task of their own choice.

(b) *Tests in which the experimental schools certainly tend to be superior, but the results are not uniformly in their favour in all tests, or else were not carried out under very satisfactory conditions.*

8. Concentration on a task which they are asked to do, but which is not immediately interesting.
9. Listening to and illustrating a passage read to them.
10. Performing certain exercises in physical training.
11. Performing a task which needs self-confidence.
12. Writing compositions (at eight years old)[1].

(c) *Those in which there is no significant difference between the two groups.*

1. Answering questions in a story read to them.
2. Carrying out a task in handwork neatly and carefully.
3. Defining words, naming pictured objects.
4. Performing certain exercises in physical training.
5. Working the answers to simple sums in arithmetic. (Both at seven and eight years old).
6. Reading (at seven and at eight years old).
7. Spelling and punctuating (at eight years old)[2].

(d) *Those in which the control groups are superior.*

1. Writing quickly and neatly (at six years old).
2. Keeping to rather unattractive rules in a game which involved following a teacher's rules for co-operating with others.

CONTACT WITH THE OUTSIDE WORLD

Another important aspect of the intellectual stimulus afforded by life in a family—one which the institution mostly lacks—is

---

[1] and [2]. These tests are taken in one pair of schools only and cannot therefore be considered as of equal importance to the tests which were given in four or more pairs of schools.

contact with the larger world outside the home, with opportunities for learning about the real life of adults.

In most institutions, there is little natural stimulus to active interests, and questionings arising from such contact with the ordinary world. Many institution children have never seen any of the basic processes of maintaining life under ordinary conditions. They have never watched mother washing, cleaning, cooking, gone shopping with her, watched the bus conductor clip the tickets, admired the driver, or gone to the pictures with father or older brother, and enjoyed all the varied and exciting life of the streets. They have no idea how an ordinary mother contrives her spending of the household money—nor learnt to manage their own pocket money. They have not had questions stirred in their minds by these interesting events and processes connected with the satisfaction of fundamental human needs, nor been stimulated to speech and to knowledge by their wish to understand these things. A colleague of mine, talking recently to an institution child, found that the child had no idea that washing ever *could* be done except in a fully equipped laundry!

It was a marked characteristic of Miss Boyce's school that she started from the children's spontaneous expression of their concern with their own experiences in the everyday life of the home and the street. By making use of these natural interests, she led them gradually forward into the more orderly and disciplined world of formal learning and the "subjects" of education. She started from the children as they were in their own narrow world, their ignorance and their knowledge, their naive interests, their fun, their halting steps towards the larger world, and their suspicions of it. She showed them what pleasure there is in learning, and what light their school learning can shed upon their personal lives. The school thus became a place to which they brought their own problems of living, and from which they took knowledge and skill and human understanding.

Now it is difficult for the large institution to take up this natural source of interest and learning—the institution constitutes a world of its own, as a rule largely artificial and cut off from the currents of life in the world outside. In an earlier quotation I have brought evidence (and the fact is a familiar one) that adolescent children who have grown up in institutions find it difficult to adapt to the ordinary demands of outside life (managing money, dealing with people, etc.) when they leave and should become independent. They have been too isolated from economic and social realities as well as too little stimulated to learn and think.

EMOTIONAL AND INTELLECTUAL DEVELOPMENT

As will have been noted, it is difficult to separate social and intellectual growth, the development (or lack of development) of character and of learning and thinking. These aspects of children's growth and of their education interact at every point. Being deprived of the chance to develop bodily and manipulative skill, and of the active means of learning and co-operating, handicaps alike the child's bodily health, emotional balance and the growth of intelligence.

Active methods of making and doing and learning are of great value in the child's character development. They help him to learn to control those natural impulses of greed and aggression and rage to which we have already referred, and to overcome the anxieties which these destructive impulses of his own arouse in him.

E.g. in considering delinquency, it is important to realize that it is not the mere lack of private possessions (although this may itself be a serious deprivation) which causes a child to steal, but often the longing for love and lack of the means of loving and creating.

The young child often shows us that he feels not only anxious about being helpless and about his own greed and aggression, but also feels doubtful about his ever becoming controlled and skilful, able to do and to create in the world as he desires. He has so little hope and confidence in his own future that he sometimes feels that the *only* way to get the good things which the grown-ups have (not merely possessions but abilities, being able to learn and understand, to create useful things, to have children of their own) is to *steal* them. Much of the actual thieving of children is an expression of these feelings. They may steal money, food, etc., but in the child's imagination these things stand not only for things to eat and money to spend, but also for the means of being powerful in well doing, in creating and giving. E.g. one boy in the top class of an infant school was discovered to have stolen money quite often; on one occasion it was a ten shilling note from his teacher's pocket. He readily confessed that he had taken it and had given it to a poor man in the street who, he said,

16

"needed it more than the teacher". This is an unusually clear instance of a fact familiar to psychologists, that the hidden motives of the child who steals may include constructive wishes as well as greed.

Another example which came my own way is that of a girl (an orphan) who had been an inmate of a Poor Law Home from early infancy until she was fifteen, when she became a servant maid in a comfortable household. She was an extremely inhibited and unresponsive personality. She did what she was asked to do but showed no open sign of feeling; no wishes or amibitions. It was, however, discovered after some months that she had appropriated various family possessions—*not* money or clothes, but family photographs and devotional books from the library of her employer! Her drawer was full of photographs of the family she lived with. Nothing could show more clearly her longing to be a member of a family and to have kind and loving parents and brothers and sisters of her own.

The child needs to feel that he *belongs*, that he is wanted and valued as a person, for what he is and what he can give. If he has the chance to develop manipulative and creative skills, to share in the social and practical life of his home, to be *active* in learning at school, he gradually comes to believe that he can contribute to others as well as take from them, can make a real return for what has been done for him when he was weak and helpless. Only *active* learning, however, and active social participation and interchange with those who love him and give him responsibility can build up in him a confidence in his own future.

SUMMARY AND CONCLUSIONS

A. ESSENTIAL NEEDS OF DEVELOPMENT

I have put forward the view that the essential needs of children, which must be met if they are to develop into useful and valuable citizens and satisfactory parents, are:

(*a*) The give and take of ordinary human affection, in a direct personal relationship with their parents or parent substitutes;

(*b*) the sense of security which can only be built up in an environment which is both stable and satisfying; e.g. one in which the persons to whom the child becomes attached do not frequently change;

(*c*) a mild steady control, relying upon positive opportunities for the child rather than upon negative injunctions;

(*d*) the companionship of other children;

(*e*) active social participation in group life, with increasing responsibility;

(*f*) the intellectual stimulus which comes from sharing in the ordinary activities of a home and being in daily contact with the world outside the home;

(*g*) opportunities for creative activity and for learning by doing.

Without these, the child's intellectual and emotional life necessarily become starved and impoverished.

B. EDUCATIONAL BEARINGS

1. If these are the needs of the child, it follows that whatever we provide as a substitute for his own home must be of such a kind as will give him the experience of family relationships, with all the emotional and intellectual stimulation and the practical activities which family life affords.

2. The evidence is clear and substantial that large institutions cannot easily perform these functions. Large institutions *tend* to impoverish the mental life, to starve the child's feelings and narrow his social development, to encourage neurotic illnesses and delinquency, and to leave the child without adequate knowledge of the outside world in which he will later have to live.

3. Smaller institutions are thus greatly preferable to larger ones. Small "grouped homes" and foster homes are far more likely to be able to meet the needs of growing children.

4. If existing institutions happen to be large, they should be broken up, as far as the daily life of the children is concerned, into small units which are capable of approximating to a family situation and creating a family atmosphere.

C. SELECTION, SUPERVISION AND TRAINING

(a) *Foster homes*

Whilst it is true that foster homes naturally provide many of the conditions we have discussed, they will only satisfy all the essential needs of the child if they are *good* foster homes. Not any and every foster home will prove helpful to the child's development —even apart from questions of gross cruelty, unkindness and neglect.

Careful *selection* is thus required by those (such as trained psychiatric social workers) who are qualified to judge, not only the material conditions, but also the personalities of the foster parents, their ways of handling children and the general atmosphere of the home.

Moreover, it is highly desirable that there should be regular *supervision* of foster homes by such properly qualified people, who will be able to help the foster parents to understand the particular children who are with them, and to deal wisely with their difficulties.

(b) *Training of staff in Institutions and Grouped Homes*

For similar reasons, it is essential that members of the staff of Institutions and Grouped Homes should be both well chosen and adequately trained. Their training should include knowledge of the psychological needs of children as well as of the requirements of bodily health, and understanding of modern methods of education. Institution staffs need to have more, not less, knowledge, understanding and skill than teachers in day schools, since they have to perform parental functions as well.

APPENDIX

The psychological state of children in Homes and Institutions—
signs to which visitors should give attention.

A. General

1. Facial expression of children; do they look happy and contented
anxious and strained, or hard and rigid? Do they return a friendly smile?

2. What is their way of speaking to the grown-ups in charge? Is this easy
and confident or formal and un-naturally polite? Are they *pleased* to see the
superintendent come in or talk to them?

3. Are they absorbed and eager in their occupations? And ready to talk
about them to visitors, if approached?

4. Are they reasonably noisy without being wild? And reasonably dirty if
at play? (Happy and active children cannot keep spotless at play—as we
know from children in our own homes. If they *are* spotless when at play, there
is something wrong.)

5. Are they quietly friendly to visitors, or either (*a*) over-demanding of
attention or (*b*) suspicious and hostile, glum or dumb?

6. Do their toys and play materials look as if they were well used? Are they
so new-looking and clean that one has the right to suspect that they are mostly
kept in the cupboards and only put out to impress visitors? (In one well-known
nursery this is surprisingly true—one cannot take it for granted that it will
not be so.)

7. What is the attitude of the children to each other? Are they reasonably
friendly and freely co-operative (without being over-polite and restrained) or
do they seem to regard other children as enemies all the time? Or are they too
subdued and nervous of what the grown-ups will say if they talk and play
freely with each other, or if they have minor quarrels?

8. How do the grown-ups speak *to* the children—with easy friendliness and
warmth, or always reproving, checking, giving orders, etc.? How do they speak
about them? Do they take an interest in them as individuals? Do they show any
awareness of the feelings and *problems* of the homeless children, or do they
regard them merely as children of bad heredity and condemn them?

9. What is the attitude of the grown-ups to such difficulties as bed-wetting,
thumb-sucking and stealing? Do they have rigid rules and harsh penalties or is
there an attempt to see the nature of the child's problem, and to allow some
latitude as regards harmless habits such as thumb-sucking? Do they approach
bed-wetting as a co-operative problem in which the child can *assist*, rather than
be treated simply as an offender and be passively punished?

10. Do the grown-ups seem to get any *pleasure* in the companionship of the
children, and happiness in their work? Or is their attitude mainly one of duty
or self-righteousness?

B. Older Children (6 years onwards)

1. They should be seen when at play without supervision. Is there a lot of
teasing and bullying? (A certain amount is more or less normal; but if there is
a great deal, this always indicates too severe a discipline at other times.)

2. Do they play in groups or with friends? Is there much solitary or aimless
standing about? Are they generally lively and active? Is there a great wildness,

with the urgent need to throw off restraint—suggesting that restraint at other times is too rigid?

3. What hobbies have they? Is there a variety of choice and enough material? Are they allowed to use odds and ends of material (and are these provided) as well as "toys"? Are they allowed to use these inventively and individually? Visitors should ask to see evidence of the children's creative play—drawing, handwork, acting, etc. This is much more valuable in itself, and more revealing, than formally ordered activities.

4. Have they any books, and are they allowed access to them? Do the books show signs of being read?

5. How is their out-of-school time planned? Have they enough chance to share in domestic activities and *not too much*? How much really free play-time do they get?

6. Do they get any experiences of life outside the institution—excursions, visits of observation, responsibility for some of the shopping, etc.?

7. Do they chatter to each other at meal-times, as they should be encouraged to do?

8. Have they their own personal possessions and a place to keep them in? Is this treated by the grown-ups with respect, as a private place, as it should be?

9. Is there a cupboard in which co-operatively owned and shared things can be kept—e.g. dressing-up properties?

10. Are they allowed to keep pets and share in the gardening?

C. YOUNGER CHILDREN (under six years)

1. Are they allowed some "messy" play with sand, water, clay, etc., as they need? These more primitive materials are essential for normal development in children from 2-5. (Some place in the garden or an outdoor shed should be provided.)

2. Is "make-believe" and imaginative play encouraged and appreciated? This should be quite unorganised and individual.

3. Do they come spontaneously to talk to the visitors? (This is the normal thing with the younger children.)

4. Have they *free* access to a variety of simple toys and play material?

5. Do they seem to be very destructive of material? A certain amount of destructiveness is normal in young children—is the attitude of the grown-ups too restrictive and condemning towards this? On the other hand, if there is a great deal of destructiveness, it means the children are starved of (a) affection and (b) the opportunity for creative and imaginative activities.

6. Have the children a chance to keep some of their constructions (railway lines, dolls' house e.g.) standing for a length of time? (It is very exasperating, and encourages destruction and aimless play, if their productions are treated with *no* respect and always have to be pulled down and put away.)

7. Is there a large dolls' house (no matter how simple and rough) in which they can play socially? This is a *most* valuable thing for social training.

INDEX OF AUTHORS

INDEX OF SUBJECTS